SIZING UP CONSCIOUSNESS

SIZING UP CONSCIOUSNESS

Towards an Objective Measure
of the Capacity for Experience

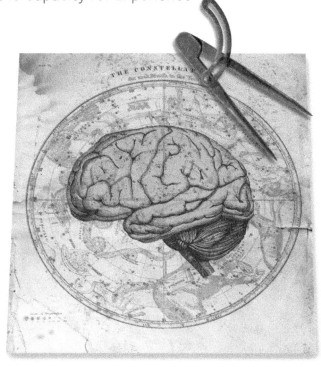

MARCELLO MASSIMINI & GIULIO TONONI

TRANSLATED BY FRANCES ANDERSON

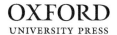

OXFORD
UNIVERSITY PRESS

OXFORD
UNIVERSITY PRESS

Great Clarendon Street, Oxford, OX2 6DP,
United Kingdom

Oxford University Press is a department of the University of Oxford.
It furthers the University's objective of excellence in research, scholarship,
and education by publishing worldwide. Oxford is a registered trade mark of
Oxford University Press in the UK and in certain other countries

Published in the United States of America by Oxford University Press
198 Madison Avenue, New York, NY 10016, United States of America

British Library Cataloguing in Publication Data

Data available

Library of Congress Control Number: 2018933552

ISBN 978–0–19–872844–3

Printed and bound by
CPI Group (UK) Ltd, Croydon, CR0 4YY

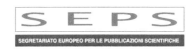

The translation of this work has been funded by SEPS
SEGRETARIATO EUROPEO PER LE PUBBLICAZIONI SCIENTIFICHE

Via Val d'Aposa 7 – 40123 Bologna – Italy
seps@seps.it – www.seps.it

PREFACE

Science has developed reliable measures for almost everything. Astronomers have learned to detect stars that are a million light-years away, but we still struggle when it comes to see the light of consciousness in the world around us. Yes, neuroscience has made enormous strides forward over the past few decades. We have a good idea now of how complicated neural circuits recognize different colors, encode memories, produce the elaborate computations that are essential for verbal communication, coordinate complicated movements, such as grasping a moving object, and much more besides. Today, we understand some of these mechanisms so well that we can replicate them in the artificial circuits of a computer. However, when we are called to answer fundamental questions about the relationships between matter and consciousness in a principled way, we become less and less confident. What is so special about a piece of flesh that can host a subject who sees light or dark? Why is the brain associated with a capacity for experience, but not the liver or the heart, as previous cultures believed? Why certain parts of the brain, but not others? Why does consciousness fade during deep sleep, while the cerebral cortex remains active? Why does it recover, vivid, and intense, during a dream? Can unresponsive patients with a functional island of cortex surrounded by widespread damage be conscious? Is a parrot that talks, or an octopus that learns and plays, conscious? Can computers be conscious? Could a system behave like us and yet be devoid of consciousness—a zombie? Here, we will not try to explain the different facets and contents of human consciousness; rather we would like to consider these broad questions in the search for a guiding principle, a general rule to size up the capacity for experience in natural and artificial entities. Most important, we wish to share a passionate scientific journey with the reader in an attempt to appreciate what is most precious within the human skull and beyond.

The journey starts in the mortuary, with a powerful experience. A medical student, attending an autopsy, is given a human brain to hold. There it lies—in the palm of his hand, and suddenly he realizes that this small, fragile object, not many hours earlier, had housed an entire universe—space, time, shapes, colors, animals, fears, hopes, the joy of a sunset. This realization comes as a shock, he is thrown into a state of confusion, and feels lost, much more so than when, as a boy, he tried to imagine the earth as a grain of sand floating in an immense, icy universe. This is how it is. Consciousness depends on a handful of neurons buzzing within the cranium; it just takes a blow to the head, a vial of general anesthetic, or just falling asleep, and the whole universe, ourselves included, disappears. Our destiny is chained to that of a small greasy machine that can seize up at any time.

There are two reasons for such a raw incipit. The first is that, frequently, accounts regarding consciousness are swamped in definitions and logical traps, and the concept becomes fuzzy, fragmented, and diluted. The student holding a brain in the palm of his hand helps to keep us on track, not to forget the fundamental question to which we have to find an answer—what makes this lump of matter, apparently not so different from the flesh of the heart and the liver—so special that it can house a subject who suffers, dreams, or simply exists? The second reason is autobiographical; we have both held a brain in our hand, albeit at different times and in different places, and neither of us has forgotten how it feels.

At the end of a journey along the boundaries of consciousness—from the cerebral cortex to the cerebellum, from wakefulness to sleep, anesthesia, and coma, from photodiodes to digital cameras, supercomputers, octopuses, dolphins, and much more besides—we will come back to the crime scene: in the mortuary with the student reappraising the brain in the palm of his hand.

Journeys benefit from a map, and our journey is no exception to the rule. The overall chart is symmetrical, with the first four chapters being dedicated to questions, the fifth offering a key to interpretation, and the last four chapters proposing answers in reverse order. The first chapter taps into existential issues that are then reconsidered in the final chapter, the second chapter poses questions of an ethical and philosophical nature that are dealt with in the eighth chapter, the third chapter examines the clinical dilemma of patients in a comatose or vegetative state, which is taken up again experimentally in the seventh chapter. The fourth chapter sets out a number of fundamental anatomical–physiological paradoxes, which are addressed in the sixth chapter. The fifth chapter introduces a theoretical principle and is the keystone of the structure. Thus, the periphery of the book (the initial and final chapters) is more speculative and evocative, whereas the arguments become increasingly stringent towards the center of the book, in line with classic scientific methodology. This book is not a typical scientific essay and we should forewarn the reader that many relevant contributions to the subject will not be mentioned—far from being exhaustive and representative of the whole field, it describes a particular scientific trajectory and a preliminary exploration of the potential practical, clinical, and ethical implications of a general principle about the nature of consciousness.

Having said this, the distinctive feature of the text is that it was written on an impulse. It is the story of a journey, told as we would tell a group of friends about a remarkable trip. After all, when it comes to conscious experience, we are all equally expert and equally naive. So, we apologize in advance for riding our hobby horses, for the digressions, the bursts of exaggerated enthusiasm, all typical of late night discussions with friends.

ACKNOWLEDGEMENTS

This book describes a preliminary attempt to translate a general principle about the nature of consciousness into practical measurements. As such, this essay is a slim reflection of a larger experimental work carried out over the last 15 years by team of researchers spread across the globe. We shared sleepless nights with Fabio Ferrarelli, Reto Huber, Steven Esser, Brady Riedner and Sean Hill while performing the first TMS-EEG measurements in sleeping brains at the University of Wisconsin. Steven Laureys and the ComaScience Group at the University of Liege made the difference; thanks to the relentless efforts of Melanie Boly (now at University of Wisconsin) Olivia Gosseries, Marie-Aurelie Bruno and Pierre Boveroux, TMS-EEG measurements could be performed for the first time at the bedside of brain-injured patients. Mario Rosanova, Silvia Casarotto, Andrea Pigorini, Matteo Fecchio, Angela Comanducci and Simone Sarasso at the University of Milan were essential: this core team developed, validated the methodology and then performed measurements in hundreds of subjects in various institution, including the Don Gnocchi Institute where, thanks to Guya Devalle, theoretical principles have meet day-to-day clinical practice. Special thanks go to Adenauer Giradi Casali (now at Universidade Federal de São Paulo, Brazil) who has been pivotal in many respects, including the design and implementation of the Perturbational Complexity Index.

The story told in this book revolves around a theory that has been developed over the years thanks to the invaluable contribution of Larissa Albantakis, David Balduzzi, Melanie Boly, Chiara Cirelli, Graham Findlay, Lice Ghilardi, Bill Marshall, Will Mayner, Masafumi Oizumi, Shun Sasai, Olaf Sporns, Nao Tsuchiya, and Christof Koch, who jump-started the science of consciousness more than two decades ago. We are also grateful to many with whom we have discussed general ideas about the nature of consciousness, providing constructive and critical comments, among them Chris Adami, Mike Alkire, Giorgio Ascoli, Bernie

Baars, Tim Bayne, Ned Block, Hal Blumenfeld, Emery Brown, Gyuri
Buszaki, Susan Blackmore, Ned Block, Jim Crutchfield, David Chalmers,
Patricia Churchland, the late Francis Crick, Antonio Damasio, Richie
Davidson, Stan Dehaene, Dan Dennett, Gerald Edelman, Karl Friston,
Stefano Fusi, Michael Gazzaniga, Mel Goodale, Allan Hobson, Tony
Hudetz, Giandomenico Iannetti, Sid Kouider, Hakwan Lau, Rodolfo
Llinas, Karlheinz Meier, Rafael Malach, Lucia Melloni, Thomas Metzinger,
Hedda Mørch, Yuval Nir, Lino Nobili, Umberto Olcese, Adrian Owen,
Brad Postle, Cyriel Pennartz, Marc Raichle, Anil Seth, Niko Schiff, Andy
Schwartz, Mavi Sanchez Vives, John Searle, Wolf Singer, Johan Fredrick
Storm, and Barry van Veen.

We are also grateful to Salvatore Vitellino at Baldini & Castoldi who
prompted us to write the first Italian version of this book, Martin Baum
at Oxford University Press who convinced us that it was a good thing
to publish it in English, Frances Anderson who translated it, Charlotte
Holloway and Sue Finlay for the excellent support in editing the final
version.

Finally, this book could be written only with the generous support
for the science that sustains it. For this, Marcello Massimini is grateful
to the McDonnell Fundation, the Brain and Mind Program of the
Canadian Institute for Advanced Research (CIFAR), the Italian Ministry
of Education, the University of Milan and the European Commission.
Special gratitude goes to the colleagues and friends involved in the
Luminous (H2020 FET) project and in the Human Brain Project through
which ideas and experiments have been developed, will further grow,
change and extend across disciplines, models and scales.

Giulio Tononi is grateful to the McDonnell Fundation, DARPA, the
NIH Director's Pioneer Award, the NIMH and NINDS, the Templeton
Foundation and the Tiny Blue Dot Foundation. His heartfelt thanks go
to the support provided by his laboratory, his department, the School of
Medicine, the UW Medical Foundation, and the University of Wisconsin.

CONTENTS

A BRAIN IN YOUR HAND

Our Planet, Our Home

Sometimes events of an extraordinary nature force us to face the actual dimension of things and leave an indelible mark. Take, for example, the astronauts of the Apollo mission, who lived the experience of setting a foot on the Moon; these men were neither poets nor philosophers, they were engineers and military pilots, men of action. They reached the Moon after years of physical training, saturated in technology, chained to rigid sequences and endless checklists, prepared for any eventuality except one . . . the mind-shattering experience of existential flight. At a certain point in time these men saw the Earth, their home planet, rising over the Moon's horizon; in that instant they became vividly aware of a new sense of the world that was difficult to share with other people. There are not many ways of expressing the power of the experience in seeing the Earth from the Moon; in fact the astronauts all use more or less the same words:

> You look back at the Earth from the Moon, and you can put your thumb up to the window and hide the Earth behind your thumb. Everything you have ever known is behind your thumb . . . (Jim Lowell)

> I put up my thumb and shut one eye, and my thumb blotted out the planet Earth. I didn't feel like a giant. I felt very, very small. (Neil Armstrong)

> The Earth reminded us of a Christmas tree ornament hanging in the blackness of space. As we got further and further away it diminished in size. Finally it shrank to the size of a marble, the most beautiful marble you can imagine. That beautiful, warm, living object looked so fragile, so delicate, that if you touched it with a finger it would crumble and fall apart. Seeing this has to change a man. (James B. Irwin)

These words may seem naive, but on reflection they are rather deep and touching. There are no attempts here to expound complicated concepts; they express simple, sincere, and genuine astonishment. There they were, men who for years had dreamed of discovering the Moon, and all of a sudden, totally unexpectedly, they discovered the Earth. They saw their planet from a distance (approximately 300 thousand km) in a new perspective. All joys, sufferings, separations, dreams, everything distilled in a colored marble that you can hide behind your thumb. Back home, the astronauts mulled over their experiences on the Moon, and talked about them on the press and on television. Even when the overwhelming impression of the first sight of the Earth from the Moon started to fade, they still remembered the strange sensation of realizing that the bright sky that spans the human tragedy and comedy is, in fact, just a thin curtain and beyond it is darkness, immense and icy. The astronauts tell how their initial feelings of anguish soon transformed into liberation, serenity, and wonder. In a split second they were able to shrug off not only the fatigue of their mission, but also the weight of ages of tormented history. Many of them tried to express the profound and constructive affection they felt for that fragile home and its inhabitants, others went so far as to suggest that this spectacular sight of the Earth from the Moon, if accessible to all (including those in positions of power), would convince mankind to make a fresh start [1].[1] Archibald McLeish, an American poet, after having seen a photograph of the Earth observed from the Moon, brought back by the Apollo mission, attempted to interpret the state of mind of the astronauts with these lines published on the *New York Times* on December 25, 1968:

> To see the earth as it truly is, small and beautiful in that eternal silence where it floats, is to see ourselves as riders on the earth together, brothers on that bright loveliness in the eternal cold, brothers who know now they are truly brothers.

Unfortunately, we cannot say that these words have had a major impact on our attitude toward the planet. However, we are left with the impression that the sight of the Earth from the Moon succeeded in putting

---

1 This cognitive shift reported by a number of astronauts is known as the overview effect; for a detailed description of this phenomenon see reference [1].

things in their correct perspective, even if for a very short time. It was like the perfect incarnation of the Copernican revolution, only 400 years later. Of course, it is difficult to describe the sensations that the astronauts felt in the exact moment when they touched the wonderful modesty of the Earth with a fingertip. Indeed, it is hardly worth the effort; certain facts unleash their power only when they hit our senses directly. In 1968 everyone knew that the Earth is round and that it lies on the periphery of an immense universe. However, knowing this is one thing, feeling it is another.

Our Brain, "Our" Home

Today much is known about consciousness and its relationship with the body. We know that it does not depend on the lungs, liver, or heart, but on a handful of neurons in the skull. It only takes a small lesion in the occipital cortex to lose the perception of color or of faces. For each of us, a traumatic brain injury or a small dose of anesthetic may obliterate the universe as we know it, including ourselves. Even if you have never experienced coma or general anesthesia, your nightly descent into sleep is your own personal experience of how delicate the relationship between consciousness and brain matter is. Every night, when we fall asleep, something changes in the way our neurons function and suddenly we do not exist anymore—to all extents and purposes, the universe as we know it dissolves into nothing. In fact, we die every night. This is extraordinary, but we don't often think about it, perhaps because we cannot experience unconsciousness. When we are unconscious, we are not present. As Epicurus pointed out long ago, there is little point in worrying about when we are not there, before birth or after death. When death comes, we go. Maybe we are not overly concerned about the annihilation of deep sleep because we know (or think we know) that the universe will come back in the space of a few seconds upon waking up. Maybe we take consciousness and our brain for granted, just as we take for granted the planet upon which we live and other things that we cannot appreciate in their true dimension because we are completely immersed in them.

If we decide to face the question of the brain-consciousness relationship straight on, the essence of the mystery eludes us. Even those who, armed with good intentions and a strong dose of curiosity, attack the vast literature that has accumulated on the subject, soon discover that it is far too easy to get lost. Start with the name itself. A disconcerting plethora of notions and definitions lie behind the term "consciousness." In certain contexts the term is used to indicate moral conscience, in others to signify awareness of self, and in others again it indicates the ability of an individual to react to a stimulus. This is just the tip of the iceberg. If we investigate further, particularly if we venture into the realms of the philosophy of mind, we soon get the impression that we must have embarked on a long and tortuous path that most likely will lead nowhere or may even turn out to be circular. It seems inevitable that we must take some philosophical stance on the relationship between matter and mind, but which? The possibilities are many, the choices seemingly arbitrary, and reference points rare—one begins to suspect that medieval scholar mulling over the proofs of God's existence must have felt similarly. Book after book, page after page, the concept of consciousness begins to disintegrate into myriads of distinctions and categories [2–4]. Who can blame us if we get discouraged? The British scholar Stuart Sutherland expressed his frustration in the introduction to his *International Dictionary of Psychology*:

> consciousness is a fascinating but elusive phenomenon: it is impossible to specify what it is, what it does, or why it evolved. Nothing worth reading has been written on it.

A harsh judgment, and you might think that it is hardly an appropriate quotation for the first chapter of a book on consciousness. It certainly expresses the despair still shared by many students and scholars alike after struggling with this subject in a nutshell. This is why we would like to open this book with an experience, rather than a definition. We will have time to sharpen the blades of logic later; for now, let us start the journey by giving free rein to our instincts.

So how can we stimulate our senses to "recognize" consciousness? Is there a way to feel the mystery of consciousness in all its power? Maybe there is one, though it does not have the heroic quality of the astronauts' experience; quite the contrary. In fact, to come to terms with consciousness, we must leave the aseptic and majestic atmosphere of outer space and step into the shoes of a medical student getting to grips with his first autopsy, trying to conquer waves of nausea in the malodorous and narrow environment of the mortuary. A first autopsy is an experience that is difficult to forget. The moment the pathologist picks up their knife, and opens the chest and the abdomen of the cadaver lying on the steel table, nearly everything that we have learned with such effort during the years of medical study falls apart before our very eyes. Those tidy organs, neatly distinct in the illustrations in the anatomy text book, are not so tidy nor are they so neatly separate; the liver isn't as brown, nor are the lungs so blue and the heart is certainly not so red. In a split second the pumps and filters, the levers and gears, all the crystalline mechanisms of physiology melt into a homogeneous mush, while wafts of the odor of decomposition penetrate our masks that have been (ineffectively) soused in aftershave. It is quite a shock to realize that we are made of such crude matter, which decomposes so rapidly. Even the most cynical medical student struggles against accepting the concept of his body being material, but it just takes one autopsy to end the struggle and this is just the beginning.

After examining the internal organs of the chest and the abdomen, the pathologist slits open the scalp, folds it back, and uses a vibrating saw to cut open the calvarium. Two or three sharp taps with a chisel and the skull cap is removed and deposited on the dissecting table with a thud. These sounds leave their mark, and echo in your ears for days just as the crash of a road accident will, if you are caught up in it. After freeing the convexity of the brain from the membranes that envelop it, the pathologist uses a spatula to lift out the frontal lobe and takes dissecting scissors to the optical nerves, the acoustic nerves, and all the other fibers that tie the brain to the cranium. One final cut to the brain stem and the cerebrum is free. The pathologist turns to the nearest student and places the brain in their palm. It is then passed from hand to hand for the students to examine it in turn. Now imagine you are next. You have a choice; you can either observe this organ like you analyzed the spleen, the liver, and the heart, then pass it on to the person standing next to you or you can stop for a moment and ponder that this damp and jelly-like mass, lying inert in your hands, was a universe as vast as your own, just a few hours ago. Everything that you are, everything that you know, that you remember, imagine, and dream is contained in an object that can be handled like any other worldly object. A thing with mass and borders. Your mind begins to whirl as it did when, as a child, you tried to imagine the immensity of the universe, and the profusion of galaxies and stars. The dizziness that you are experiencing may even be stronger than what the astronauts felt when watching the small Earth setting behind the Moon. Holding a brain in your hand is an overwhelming experience that, in the blink of an eye, erases all the habits, philosophical positions, definitions, and logical traps that stand between us and the mystery of consciousness. It is almost an initiation, one that any scholar interested in consciousness should go through. A simple question seems to spring spontaneously from the nerves of the hand holding the brain, clamoring for an answer. What makes this object so different from the rest? What makes it so special?

There, standing in front of the dissection table, you don't ask how it is possible that brain matter can feed the contorted flames of self-reflection, nor do you feel the need to understand how it manages to produce the perception of a scene from one of Brueghel's crowded paintings. You have just examined the liver and heart, so you simply ask how it is possible that this tofu-like organ, which weighs 1.5 kg if that, can host a subject who can see light or just pure dark. Why the brain, but not the other organs? Of course, you are a model student and you remember that the brain generates electric signals; but just a moment! So, does the heart. Of course! the brain is composed of tens of billions of neurons and trillions of synapses . . . ah, but within the brain the cerebellum has even more neurons and synapses than the cerebrum, and it has nothing to do with consciousness. Then you remember that during the physiology course they told you that, in certain phases of sleep, the brain isolates itself temporarily from the nerves that connect it to the outside world and starts dreaming—a vivid, colorful, riotous universe, generated entirely from within. You are struck by the thought that this fragile mass of tissue lying here in your hand could dream, if it were drenched in the right solution of sugar and oxygen, and while you are still standing there trying to collect your thoughts, your neighbor nudges you; it is time to pass the brain on. This intense and tangible mystery unfolds in little over 1 min, but what power it can have!

As students, we both had a similar experience in the mortuary. Both of us are convinced that the effect of holding a brain, feeling its texture and weight, is not unlike hiding the Earth behind your thumb at 300 thousand km. It is a sublime experience, in the philosophical and literary sense of the term; it is both a source of mental anguish and liberation. In the first place, it is disturbing to have to attribute the perfection, beauty, and integrity of what we can conceive and perceive to such a humble object; a small greasy machine whose working parts will, sooner or later, break down and melt. This cannot be right; we are much more than this! A glance at the cadaver on the dissection table, his open eyes, however, is enough to convince us that not long before, this body was a being who could see, hear, feel, and think, from the smallest to the grandest though, just as we can. The astronauts saw the extraordinary richness of the world in a tiny colored marble suspended in space. We grasped the borders of the humble matter that contains anything that can be experienced. During the autopsy, we have held the forbidden fruit and there is no going back. Innocence is lost. We must swear that we will not accept pseudo-solutions and will take nothing for granted. We are aware that a valid scientific explanation of consciousness must stand up to the test of facts and measures, but we also know that it must stand up to the test of our senses and the judgment of our instinct. If one day, holding a brain in our hand will be much more a revelation and much less of a challenge, we will have somehow succeeded.

CHAPTER 2

ZOMBIES AND DOLLS

W e have just stepped into the shoes of a young medical student staring at a grey, soft mass in the palm of his hand. Just like Hamlet musing on the skull of Yorick, the court jester, he is deeply disturbed by the juxtaposition of the richness of being and the poverty of matter. Both our student and Hamlet are faced with a tangible and unavoidable question. What is so special about this small and seemingly modest object? There must be something! For many, this question will remain unanswered. Any attempt to *understand* the physical weight of consciousness is doomed to failure, and the miracle of how the brain produces consciousness will remain just that, a miracle that requires an act of faith like the miracle of water being transformed into wine [5].[1] The young student is obviously not in the mood to give up, but for the time being, let skepticism take the upper hand. In fact, skepticism has deep historical and philosophical roots, and an interesting rationale that is well worth exploring.

A Philosopher's Doubt

Dualism, a line of philosophical thought that still poses tough challenges to a scientific approach to consciousness, has a long history that started, at least officially, with Descartes. The French philosopher held that consciousness has nothing to do with the physical world [6]. In his view, the fact that we can have a clear and distinct idea of ourselves as thinking beings, completely different from the idea we have of our body as a material extension, is irrefutable proof that consciousness and the mind are

---

1 The effective analogy of the water of the physical brain turned into the wine of consciousness was introduced by the British Philosopher Colin McGinn [5].

two separate entities. The attribute that defines matter is its extension—the fact that it occupies space, and so can be measured and explained in scientific terms. The attribute which defines the mind, on the other hand, is thought, which being immaterial in nature cannot be measured. These two substances are ontologically different and the insurmountable barrier between material and mental substances, between the *res extensa* and the *res cogitans*, lies at the heart of the dualist standpoint.

Centuries after Descartes, this position still enjoys support, because it appears simple and easy to grasp, and also because it complies with the natural human reluctance to be considered on a level with the other objects on the planet. On a closer look, however, the dualist approach also has its share of contradictions and problems. For example, how is it possible that something that affects the body (a burn, for example), provokes a response at mental level (the sensation of pain)? How is it possible for a thought to result in the physical movement of an arm or leg? How can a chemical anesthetic or a physical trauma pause our existence for hours or even years? Even the most hard-boiled dualist has to admit that there is a connection between matter and mind somewhere, but where? Descartes solved the question by proposing the pineal gland (epiphysis), a small structure situated in the center of the brain, as an exclusive place in which mind and matter could interact. This solution did not go down well in the 16th century and obviously does not pass muster in today's more sophisticated environment. However, even if we smile and discard Descartes' attempt as ingenuous, the fact remains that there is still no agreement as to where two ontologically separate substances might interact.

This said, today's dualists appear to be less concerned with finding a solution to the mystery of the mind–matter relationship than with underlining the limits of the scientific approach to the problem. We are not going to find the place where matter becomes experience, simply because it does not exist. Consciousness is one thing and matter is another, and science has no way of making the two become one. This is an important point, which deserves serious pondering.

Philosophical Zombies

Believe it or not, contemporary philosophy often uses zombies to illustrate the dualist perspective. These philosophical zombies (also known as p-zombies) came to notice thanks to the Australian philosopher David Chalmers [7] and, of course, have no relation to the Creole undead evoked by Caribbean witch doctors or to the partially decomposed corpses that chase people in B-movies. Philosophical zombies are well-mannered, respectable, and undistinguishable from the man in the street as far as their behavior is concerned. No medical or psychological examination will reveal any dissimilarity between a human being and a philosophical zombie. The only difference is that the philosophical zombie is totally devoid of subjective experience. If they touch a blistering hot surface they will snatch their hand back, will scream and swear like a trooper, but in point of fact, they do not feel pain. They feel nothing. According to many contemporary philosophers, the very fact that it is possible to think of a creature that from the material point of view is like us, but does not have any subjective experience (Figure 2.1), indicates that consciousness cannot be inferred from physical properties. These zombies don't eat human flesh, but they still manage to terrorize conferences dedicated to the science of consciousness, where they are evoked by witch-doctors camouflaged as cultivated scholars to embarrass and paralyze naïve speakers.

As often happens in philosophical debate, every argument or thought experiment has a counter-argument or -experiment. Of course, zombies are no exception to this. For example, it has been argued that the very possibility of the existence of a philosophical zombie conflicts with our certainty that we are sentient beings [8]. Indeed, if the zombies function as we do, surely they, too, will have this same certainty. If they can entertain this false belief, who can say that we ourselves are not mistaken when we maintain that we are thinking beings? As per this counter-argument, assuming that it is absurd to throw doubt on our subjective experience, philosophical zombies are neither possible nor conceivable. Several books and dozens of articles have been written on this subject, but who is right and who is wrong? This is an example of the circular traps that we would like to avoid, so we will take this argument no further. As we stated in Chapter 1, "A Brain in Your Palm," we prefer to keep our feet on the ground, rather than experience the frisson of logical disorientation; hence, we will now attempt to reformulate the problem of the zombies in a different way.

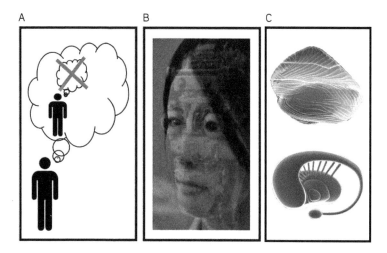

Figure 2.1 Different kinds of zombies. (A) A graphic representation of a philosophical zombie: the possibility of conceiving a being that is physically and behaviorally identical to us, but does not possess conscious experience. (B) Actroid-F, the android developed by the University of Osaka and a forerunner of the digital zombie. The sensors and the activators are visible under the artificial silicon "skin." (C) Two biological zombies, which reside in the cranium—the cerebellum (above) and the basal ganglia (below).

Figure 2.1c Upper: Source: CLIPAREA l Custom media/Shutterstock.com.

Figure 2.1c Lower: Source: decade3d—anatomy online/Shutterstock.com.

Digital Zombies

Take one of the latest generation smartphones, connect it to Internet, and download an app with a search engine, and software for voice recognition and synthesized speech; now you have a small object that can respond to many questions, remind you of your appointments, and suggest a good restaurant close by that fits in with your past choices of menu and price bracket. The voice of such devices is becoming so friendly and helpful that you might soon catch yourself saying thank you to your digital assistant! Of course, until now it has always been perfectly natural to attribute consciousness to someone who listens to us and then replies, but a smartphone certainly isn't conscious. Sure, it may fool us for a few seconds, and then only when we are distracted, but of course we can tell.

However, imagine what might happen if something rather more powerful were to be placed between the microphone and the voice synthesizer, such as Watson, the 3-million dollar IBM computer with 2880 processors and 16 terabytes RAM that can process 500 GB/s. In 2011, Watson was invited to participate in the popular American television quiz show, Jeopardy [9]. The game consisted of pressing a button before the other participants, then answering a series of questions correctly. These questions were quite difficult to interpret as they were formulated like crossword clues, playing on words and double meanings. For three episodes, which attracted huge audiences, Watson challenged the two champions of the program. The computer played large sums of money when it was sure to win, just a few dollars when it was not sure of the answer, and didn't press the button when it did not have the answer at all. Its monitor even blushed when it made a mistake. In the end it won, much to the disappointment of the two human champions and the delight of the public, who had become its ardent fan in just a few hours. Poor Watson didn't know it had won, however; in fact, Watson never experienced anything about anything. When a modern computer responds correctly to our input, when it produces an error message, crashes, or reboots, it does not understand the meaning or significance of what it is saying or doing; there is a consensus on this, even among the audience who instinctively attributed to Watson plenty of human ambitions and emotions.

In fact, it is unlikely that the software of the supercomputer would have passed the exam that computers should "dream" of passing—the Turing Test, introduced in 1950 by Alan Turing [10], the British mathematician who influenced the outcome of World War II by deciphering the German codes and considered to be the father of information technology. The Turing Test was constructed around the question "how can we know if a computer understands what it says?" Turing devised a pragmatic solution, based on the following principle: a machine can think and understand what is said to the extent that it can sustain a conversation that is indistinguishable from a conversation between two human beings. In practical terms, the Turing Test consists of a conversation held at a distance between two terminals, with an exchange of comments such as we have today when opening a conversation using Skype or Messenger. If, at a certain point, it is clear that the respondent on the other end is a machine and not a human being, then the machine has failed. If the machine dupes us into believing that we are chatting with a human being, the machine has passed the test.

There is no doubt that Watson, who could have beaten anybody at "Jeopardy!" would have tripped up in the early phases of a simple chat. The first exchanges, "How are you?," "How are things?," would not have constituted a problem, and it might even have been able to respond to specific questions, even difficult ones, but there would have been something "off." After a while, we would have had the irritating impression that the interlocutor on the other end of the line was not paying attention, or had not grasped the context of the conversation. It would not have been long before an absurd misunderstanding or a totally irrelevant answer would have revealed the non-human identity of the other party to the conversation.

While it is likely that Watson would not pass the Turing Test, better hardware running smarter software may soon do that, even in a face-to-face encounter. Imagine a much more powerful supercomputer (even in 2011 Watson was only ranked 94th) and plug it inside a futuristic version of Actroid-F, the gynoid robot developed by the University of Osaka. This humanoid machine replicates the movements and facial expressions of a young Japanese girl, including tics and emotions (Figure 2.1B), through a system of sensors and actuators [11]. It is perfectly conceivable that a mix of microprocessors, optical fibers, sensors and compressed air activators, microphones, and speech recognition software, covered in soft silicone, may one day dupe an unwary interlocutor into thinking it is human for a fairly long period of time. The futuristic android will call on a powerful combination of calculation, speed, machine learning algorithms, and access to immense databases to produce a fluid and appropriate conversation. In a face-to-face encounter, we may be a little perplexed by some inaccuracies, but it is likely that we will attribute them to intriguing cultural differences and, enchanted by the gentle ways of this exotic companion, we may even propose a romantic place for dinner. Then, just as we are about to shyly suggest our favorite restaurant, our enhanced version of Actroid-F may pull the mask off, leaving us with the humiliating sensation of having been fooled by a fancy doll.

After all, on close reflection, it is quite easy to see how a black box, which provides appropriate responses to any question, does not necessarily house someone who understands. This can best be illustrated by the Chinese room thought experiment conceived by John Roger Searle

[12]. Pretend you are in a huge box, armed with pen and paper, and an exhaustive catalogue in which all the questions that can be formulated in Japanese kanji are each associated with the correct answers, also written in Japanese kanji.[2] There is a hole in the side of the box through which someone on the outside passes you slips of paper on which are written questions. You painstakingly consult the catalogue, find the question which corresponds visually to the one written on the paper you have received, and copy down the answer. You provide the correct answer every time, even though you do not know Japanese and have understood nothing, neither the question nor the answer. You have simply followed the instructions to the letter. This will probably be the system the android will follow, just much faster, to converse with you in the future. Millions of processors will consult an exhaustive catalogue of possible questions and answers, and provide the most appropriate answer at the speed of light. This is perfectly conceivable. Searle's insight was to put ourselves in the place of the computer in order to understand that, even if we could manipulate the symbols perfectly, we would understand and feel nothing.

This is when we are struck by a thought. What if our brain, too, is just an expert manipulator of symbols? Just as the silicon microprocessors exchange digital symbols along optical fibers, so the neurons in our brain exchange electrical impulses through microscopic cables composed of fat and proteins. Could they do this without understanding anything, without feeling anything, without "being" anyone? We hope that this digression into the world of digital zombies has helped to clarify the doubt expressed by the philosophical zombies. In all cases, the most remarkable zombies live elsewhere. Indeed, they are much closer.

Zombies Within Our Skulls

In 2001, Christof Koch and Francis Crick [13] published a note in the journal *Nature* called "The zombie within." In the note, they argued that our brain contains a large number of "zombie systems," whose hallmarks are efficient sensorimotor behavior and immediate, rapid action.

---

2 Here, to be consistent with the nationality of Actroid-F, we play with Japanese writing, rather than with Chinese characters as in the original formulation.

Every waking day, we live in close contact with faithful and silent servants of whose presence we are mostly unaware. We don't notice them because they do what they do in the dark, far from the flame of consciousness, but they are there. In fact, we often teach them to do what they do. Imagine (or remember) the first lesson on the piano. You can take nothing for granted, you must make a conscious effort in every movement—how to sit on the stool, the correct posture, how to place your hands on the keyboard, how to move your fingers. You touch the keys—your performance is slow, staccato, labored. As time goes by, you become more proficient and your performance improves. The learning process that a human being undertakes is both tangible and extraordinary, but what is truly amazing is that once you have learnt the complicated motor sequences that in the initial phases absorbed every iota of concentration, they cease to appear on your "radar." You no longer have to consciously think about these sequences. They become so automatic they cease to exist and your consciousness, liberated from the fetters of the motor sequences, can apply itself to how the music should be interpreted. It is almost as if a mysterious entity in the subconscious, which moves surely and swiftly, much more surely and swiftly than we ourselves do, has taken over. Someone or something is playing the pianoforte in your place, and is playing it well. Music teachers understand this phenomenon perfectly, and at a certain point tell their students "let your fingers play, don't think about it," and one of those faithful zombies that live in the cerebrum will execute the notes fluidly, without hesitation, and without making even the slightest mistake. If you try to take back control of the motor sequence, then inevitably your performance slows down or you hit the wrong notes. This is because your inner zombie has become much better at playing the piano than you, and does not appreciate interference, only indications of a very general nature. The pianoforte is just one example, but there are many others—when your hands and feet automatically work accelerator and brake, to maintain the correct distance from the vehicle in front, while you chat to your companions; when you find the right words at the right time, with the right inflection and meaning, while in reality you only have a vague idea of what you want to say; when your skis navigate bumps in the snow, while you admire the view of distant peaks. In all these instances you have to thank an unconscious entity that works for you.

Where do these scrupulous, devoted servants live? The answer comes from clinical neurology. It is probable that there are zombies all over the place in our brain, but certain types of cerebral lesion have shown that the majority are to be found in two neural structures: the cerebellum, in the posterior cranial fossa and the basal ganglia, a voluminous mass of neurons drowned in the depths of the cerebral hemispheres (Figure 2.1C). If one of these two structures is destroyed or degenerates, life becomes very difficult. We become painfully conscious of every gesture, particularly of those of which we were previously hardly aware. When an inner zombie dies, we suddenly become aware of the importance of the work it did for us. Even the most banal tasks, such as grasping a glass of water, become arduous. Distances must be calculated, movements measured, the hand has to open at the right time and be closed with the correct amount of pressure—too strong a grip and we break the glass, too weak and the glass slips through our fingers. With all these complications, errors are inevitable [14]. Many, too many, of the tasks that were carried out by the zombie now have to come under our control [15]. The luxury of that light unconscious management that we took for granted is gone for good and the resulting overload is impossible to manage. If the cerebellum is destroyed, even shaking a friend's hand is a complicated task, and driving a car or learning to play a musical instrument becomes extremely hard.

We become aware of these zombies when they disappear, but also when they malfunction and stop collaborating. Tourette syndrome, commonly known as Tourette's, is a disorder of the basal ganglia characterized by forms of behavior, some of which are quite complex, that the person is unable to control [16]. Symptoms include tics, such as spontaneous exclamations, sometimes socially inacceptable (coprolalia), repeating what others have said (echolalia), and repetition of one's own words (palilalia), although blinking and throat clearing are the most common symptoms. Persons with Tourette's may suddenly execute complicated dance steps or pirouettes. They often have a high IQ, but face great challenges in life because they are not always able to control what they say and do. It is as if a mischievous alien, residing in the depths of their brain, takes over their body, and makes them move and speak out of character.

These zombies are more than just a logical possibility. They are composed of neurons, synapses, and circuits; they live in our brain, they speak, walk, and do other complicated things without sparking the flame of consciousness. Why? What is the mysterious ingredient that is missing in their make-up? As was argued by Koch and Crick, the existence of zombie systems raises two questions. First, why aren't we just big bundles of unconscious fast zombie agents? Why bother with consciousness, which takes almost half a second to set in? Second, what is the difference between the neuronal circuits that make up zombie agents and those that support conscious experience? Addressing these kinds of questions is exactly what scientists can and should do. Indeed, when Crick and Koch jump-started the whole field of the neuroscience of consciousness and shattered the unwritten rule that forbade scientists to even mention consciousness as a subject worthy of serious inquiry, they did so precisely because they knew how to frame their questions in concrete, experimental terms. The zombies in the brain seem to be the incarnation of the abstract doubts of the philosopher. We can touch them and study them, but until we have understood them, skepticism is more than justified.

A Neuroscientist's Doubt

So, what can neuroscientists say about consciousness? After all, they are in close contact with damp biological matter every day. One thing is certain; they will not have an inferiority complex with regard to philosophers. Physiology has been extremely successful in explaining how the heart pumps blood, and how the liver and the kidneys filter and purify it. Over the last 50 years, neurophysiology and the neurosciences in general have literally exploded and our knowledge of the brain has increased exponentially. An untold quantity of data accumulates each day in thousands of neuroscience departments and continues to grow. Teams of students, graduates, postgraduates, and researchers slave daily on experiments and data, using increasingly powerful instruments. Ten years ago, it was difficult to record brain activity with more than 20 sensors; now we can cover the brain with hundreds of electrodes. In the past, a university purchasing a magnetic resonance imaging (MRI) scanner made the national headlines, today you can find scanners in almost any basement, where the anatomy and the metabolism of the human brain can be recorded with millimeter precision in vivo. Not to mention the electron microscopes, which can capture the detail of a synapsis with Angstrom-level spatial resolution (0.0000007 mm), two-photon imaging techniques, optogenetics, and the like.

There are scholars in the field of neuroscience who have dedicated their lives to understanding the workings of a single molecule, expressed in a particular class of neurons, located in a particular structure of the brain, anywhere between the periphery of the spinal cord to the more noble areas of the association cortex. The competition between laboratories is fierce; no angle of the brain forest has been left in its virgin state, researchers have marked every tree, colonized and cultivated every millimeter. You are curious about the structure of the cells in the eye of a fruit fly? You want to know about the neurons of the human cerebral cortex that are specialized in recognizing Jennifer Aniston [17]? The stands of the Annual Meeting of the Society for Neuroscience, a bustling scientific fair, which attracts at least 30,000 scientists every year, have it all.

All this effort has been rewarded with results. Neurophysiologists are revealing the neural mechanisms that control how we grasp an object— the programing of motor sequences, anticipatory postural adjustments, the perfect coordination of the limbs, fine control of the force needed from the finger muscles. These are complex mechanisms that are not yet completely understood, but it is just a question of time, there is nothing mysterious or unfathomable. Similarly, they are demystifying much of the visual system's working—from the receptive field of the rods and cones of the retina to the mechanisms of motion detection higher up in the cortical hierarchy. These successes are replicated for hearing, smell, touch, and much more.

In principle, it will soon be possible to draw a precise diagram of the auditory and visual systems, of the sense of touch, and the circuits dedicated to motor planning and control. With time and patience, we will be able to piece together a detailed diagram of the circuits in the brain and reconstruct them one-by-one, just as a counterfeiter might replicated complicated objects—such as a digital camera, car, or a military airplane—based on a stolen blueprint. The chances are that we will end up with a tangled mass of artificial neurons that behave just like the real ones, but will this bring us closer to the solution of the mystery of consciousness? Not necessarily. Let us see why, again using a tangible example.

The scientists of Lausanne Polytechnic have been working for years on a scientific enterprise without precedent, the Blue Brain project. A team of researchers from a number of fields—physicists, biologists, physiologists and computer scientists—are reproducing everything that is known about the brain into a supercomputer simulation: molecules, synapses, the electrical properties of different neurons and their patterns of connectivity, with the objective of reproducing entire areas of the cortex and, finally, the entire brain. By the end of 2006, the project had achieved its first objective, the reconstruction of a simplified cortical column. This is a cylindrical structure, about 2 mm high and 0.5 mm in diameter, which is thought to represent the fundamental functional unit for the cerebral cortex. Artificial cortical columns are much bigger than biological columns; they are housed in a supercomputer that takes up a large room. A few years ago, the project reached another landmark, the detailed simulation of a portion of the rat's somatosensory cortex containing about 30,000 simulated neurons (of 200 different types) connected by 40 million synapses [18]. This is, without doubt, the most complete simulation to date of a piece of excitable brain matter. In the years to come, petaflops of computer power and smart algorithms will grow this chunk of digital cortex further. Indeed, the project, which represents a fantastic scientific adventure, can count on generous financing and is very ambitious. Its goal is to create a virtual mouse brain with hundreds of millions of neurons and, ultimately, simulate the human brain.

Now, let us fast-forward a few decades and suppose that the empirical data and mathematical models used to reconstruct virtual neurons, their biophysical properties, and their connections are correct and complete, that their activity can be simulated in real time on a powerful supercomputer that can fit inside an artificial head, and that two artificial eyes, two ears, a nose, two nimble robotic hands, two legs and a smooth digital vocalizing system have been plugged in. Now, imagine that you have been asked to sign a rather peculiar contract, which establishes that at a certain point in your existence, when your body starts to show the first irrefutable signs of deterioration or the signs of an untreatable disease, you will hand over your biological brain to a group of scientists. You will be allowed to say your last goodbyes to family and friends, then the scientists will anesthetize you, extract your brain and record its activity with billions of sensors. They will cut it into sections, take photographs of it with the electronic microscope and analyze it thoroughly. Finally, all your neurons, their biophysical properties, and their connections will be uploaded and simulated by virtual neurons implemented by the super-computer inside the head of your new artificial body. Every last detail will be simulated faithfully, the synapses of the hippocampus, where your most vivid memories are stored, the circuits of the amygdala where the events and conditioning of your own unique life have carved out fears that you have never confessed to yourself, and so on. Trains of neuronal spikes will run incessantly across the simulation, millions per seconds, replicating the coding and the computations of your original brain and all this will rely on silicon chips, which are impervious to viruses, tumors, or heart attacks, and do not suffer the effects of the passing of time. The "silicon you" will behave exactly as you always did, and everybody will think that inside the new body there is you—the same old you—with all your idiosyncrasies, obsessions, and your few endearing traits. The contract promises you the digital immortality of your brain's activity in exchange for renouncing a few months of biological life. It lures you with the promise of watching your children grow up, enjoying their successes, and offering a helping hand when needed, of continuing to see your friends, and even the option of asking to switch off the whole thing when you have had enough.

The stakes are high, very high, and the goal is to turn one of man's greatest dreams, immortality, into reality. There are doubts, however, just as strong as the stakes are high. How many people would actually sign a similar contract? It is quite possible that not even the most optimistic of scientists, the most hard-boiled materialist and anti-dualist would put his signature to this agreement, when his time comes. Not in the name of moral qualms, but because an inner voice whispers incessantly, "Who says that being a machine that simulates exactly the activity of all your neurons is the same as being you? Who says that scientists have understood the relevant properties of the brain that have to be reproduced? What if the spatial–temporal grain at which the simulation runs is not the right one? What if the secret of consciousness is tucked away in a sub-atomic detail of the functioning of neuronal membranes? What if, instead, the relevant processes occur through unknown interactions that extend beyond my brain? Maybe, it is a particular chemical aspect of the biological matter, which cannot be reproduced on a silicon chip? Am I trading my last conscious days for a reincarnation as an eternal zombie? Do not sign! Put that pen down and go and hug your family one more time!"

The bottom line is that we totally trust science when it is a question of substituting vital organs, such as hearts and kidneys, with artificial devices, but when it comes to the brain, that is a different ball game altogether. Why are we so reluctant? Because we have a niggling suspicion that however much we know about those billions of neurons in our head and how they function, we are no closer to a scientific explanation of how the brain generates subjective experience. This is the doubt that troubles physiologists, who feel rather like the early astronomers with their detailed descriptions and charts of the movements of the celestial bodies, but who had no idea as to whether those movements were dictated by a general law. When all is said and done, our doubts, and the doubts of the physiologist and the philosopher, may share the same rational root. When it comes to the relationships between consciousness and the brain, we have described a lot, but we lack principles.

CHAPTER 3

BRAIN ISLANDS

Now we leave the morgue, the digital dolls, and the zombies, and move to the intensive care unit (ICU), where living human beings fluctuate between consciousness and unconsciousness, and where sometimes the flame of experience burns unseen on brain islands lost in a sea of neural dissolution. Here, among the tubes and drip-feeds, artificial lungs, and monitors, the way we pose the question changes, but the question itself remains the same.

Bad Awakening

How do we know a fellow human being is conscious? In the normal run of things, the question doesn't even arise. Unless we are really into philosophical zombies, we just assume that others are conscious beings—we are similar physically, so we will be similar in having subjective experiences. If your friend has nodded off on the settee in front of the television, or seems to be lost in a world of his own, you can ask something along the lines of "are you with us?" and a gesture of the hand or a grunt is all that is needed to reassure you that he has not "lost his senses." A doctor uses much the same method to evaluate the level of consciousness of a patient who has just been given a dose of anesthetic in the operating theater, or of a man arriving in the Emergency Ward with his eyes closed and his face covered in blood. In cases such as these, the doctor asks the patient to open his eyes, say his name, say where he is, and clench his right or left fist. If the patient responds, he is conscious. If there is no response, the doctor will try exerting pressure on the palm of the patient's hand, or on the nail bed to elicit pain. If there is still no response, the patient is considered to be unconscious. So, the fundamental criterion for establishing the conscious existence of another human being is whether he is able to respond to stimuli and commands. This method normally works well, but not always.

> […] that grey and silent abyss suddenly takes on a green hue, hazy at first, but which gradually comes into focus; at the same time, I can hear faint noises in the distance, now they are coming nearer and I can hear them more clearly. Where am I? Ah, of course, the operation! I am having difficulty in getting my thoughts together, but yes, this is it, the operation and now I can see the curtain through half-closed eyelids. The first impression is that it is happening to someone else, indifference mixed with stupor; but then I am seized with an impelling desire to move. I make a superhuman effort, but fail: not because I feel tied down, but because I don't have a body to move. I am just a brain floating in a void and somewhere I have a mouth, blocked by something that stops me using it, that prevents me from calling out. Everything else has just disappeared, dissolved! As soon as I realize that they are operating on me, and I am awake, damnably awake even if I can't feel anything, panic explodes. But this is a strange sort of panic, logical, ascetic, without emotion, without heartbeats because I haven't a heart, without pain because I haven't a body, without anxiety because what is happening has been decided by someone else. It is mental panic, empty panic; an anguished delirium from which there is no escape. I have no idea how long it lasts, but to me it is an eternity. I pray that it will end, I want to do something to make it end, but I don't know what. Then, finally, everything fades out …

This first-person account by a patient who accidently recovered consciousness during an operation was published in a specialized scientific journal [19]. As chance would have it, the patient was himself an anesthesiologist, a doctor well-accustomed to playing with powerful drugs and with the consciousness of other people. The unfortunate anesthesiologist suddenly awakens with the crisp realization that he's still undergoing a surgical intervention. He feels a desperate urge to move and shout to his colleagues to let them know that he is conscious, but he can't. He is fully paralyzed and artificially ventilated though a tube stuck in his throat. The agony lasts for an undefined period (presumably, a few minutes) until an additional dose of anesthetic knocks him back into unconsciousness.

Regaining consciousness during an operation, technically called "anesthesia awareness," is a fairly rare occurrence. Approximately one patient in 1000 reports having been conscious during an operation that required general anesthetic [20, 21]. Fortunately, it is extremely rare (though not impossible) for the patient to feel pain, as the patient is also given analgesic compounds before and during the operation. Even so, it is a traumatic experience that may have serious psychological consequences [22, 23]. The anguish and the trauma are to be attributed mainly to the total paralysis that the subject experiences upon regaining awareness [24]. Immediately after administering the general anesthetic and before the surgeon starts to operate, the patient receives an injection of neuromuscular blocking drugs (NBDs), which completely block the transmission of electric impulses from the nerve endings to the muscles. This block prevents the muscles from generating violent reflex contractions during the various phases of the operation, although it also impedes the patient from expanding his chest autonomously, so air is pumped into the lungs through a tube to support ventilation. Normally, patients are not aware of this as they lose consciousness just a few seconds after receiving the anesthetic and regain it only when they are back on the ward. When everything goes as planned, between the lights in the operating theater, which seem to flicker and collapse before slipping into darkness, and the anxious faces of your loved ones in the ward, you just cease to exist.

It is still not clear why some patients regain consciousness on the operating table, in spite of having received an adequate dose of anesthetic [25]. The problem is that it is difficult for the anesthesiologist to detect the recovery of consciousness during surgery [26]. The total paralysis makes it impossible for the patient to communicate with the medical team; he is forced to witness as the operation proceeds. He is present, but cannot make anyone aware of the fact. He can see, but cannot act. He can hear, but cannot communicate. He is a conscious prisoner in his own skull. Probably, the closest thing to being buried alive. In Victorian times, the fear of such a terrifying possibility led to a plethora of "safety coffin" designs: coffins equipped with complicated devices, whereby a cord was tied round the corpse's wrist and chest was linked to lamps, bells, and flags on the surface of the tomb; any movement would set off a system of visual and acoustic alarms (Figure 3.1). For a small fee, these curious contraptions could be rented and installed in the coffin for a few days or even a few weeks. As far as we know, none of the scrupulous customers of these safety coffins ever recovered from death, and there are no records on hand to tell us how many men and women were, in fact, erroneously buried alive. We can only hope none or, at the worst, very few.

Returning to the operating theater, however, there are reasons to suspect that the number of people who regain consciousness during an operation is more than 1 in 1000. This suspicion is raised by the application of a simple technique that is very reminiscent of the safety coffins, the isolated forearm technique (IFT) [27]. This method leaves an open channel between the patient's brain and the anesthesiologist in the operating theater. In the IFT, a padded cuff/tourniquet is applied to the forearm before the NBD is injected, so that the muscles in the forearm are not paralyzed and can be used to communicate with the medical team. Even though the rest of his body is blocked and he is unable to speak, the patient is still able to clench and unclench his non-paralyzed fist. The IFT is rather laborious and is not always suitable for general surgery, but has provided some interesting data. The patients who clench their fists on the operating table when the anesthetist asks "are you still with us?" may be much more numerous than those who later recall that they were conscious during the operation, maybe 1 in 10 as opposed to 1 in 1000 [26]. Whether the IFT actually reflect the persistence of consciousness or, rather, an automatic reaction is still a matter of debate [28], yet anesthesia-induced amnesia [29] may certainly contribute to the underestimation of intraoperative awareness. In all cases, consciousness does not need to be remembered in order to exist; for example, we are acutely conscious of what we are doing during a drinking spree, even if the next day we have absolutely no recall of what happened. Who would accept to endure or inflict a minute of unsupportable pain, even if given a promise that afterwards there would be no memory of it?

Fortunately, those patients who do suffer intraoperative awakening can count on the fact that, however distressing it may be at the time, the nightmare will end: muscular paralysis is reversible and once they leave the operating theater, they will either have blissfully forgotten their ordeal or will be able to forcefully explain to the surgeons what they have been through. Intraoperative awakening remains a problem for anesthesiologists, but above all it is a general admonition that we cannot afford to ignore. There are cases in which consciousness is present, desperately and intensely present, but cannot be detected from the outside. This throws doubt on our ability to promptly recognize consciousness in our fellow human beings, a doubt that becomes anguish when we are faced with patients who have emerged from coma, but lie immobile and glassy-eyed, for months or even years.

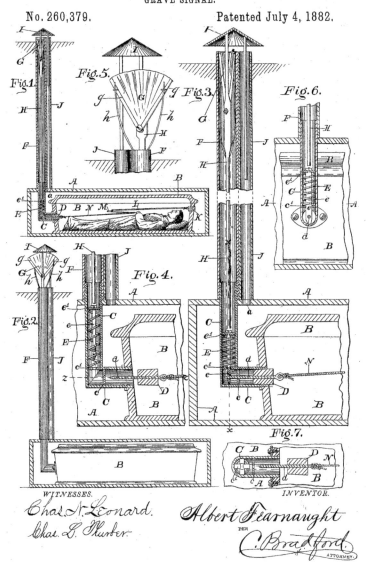

(No Model.)

A. FEARNAUGHT.
GRAVE SIGNAL.

No. 260,379.

Patented July 4, 1882.

WITNESSES.

Chas. N. Leonard.
Chas. G. Thurber.

INVENTOR.

Albert Fearnaught
PER
C. Bradford
ATTORNEY.

Surviving Coma

Coma comes from the Greek, and its original meaning is "deep sleep;" indeed, a coma closely resembles sleep. The patient lies motionless with his eyes closed, but whereas, in true sleep, all that is needed to wake a person is a gentle shake, no external stimuli will wake the person in a coma [30, 31]. In some cases, painful stimuli may provoke a brief reflexive reaction, but nothing more. The ancient Greeks used the word coma both for the heavy "comatose" sleep that follows a night on the town, and the sleep from which there is no awakening, the sleep that Penelope begged for, distraught for the absence of Ulysses. Until about 50 years ago, that just about described it. If a person who fell into a coma did not recover contact with the world shortly after, he slid into that deadly sleep from which there is no return. The state of coma is typically associated with traumatic, vascular, toxic, or anoxic distress of the brain, including a phylogenetically ancient structure that is situated deep in the skull and connects the cerebrum to the spinal cord—the brain stem [30]. The brainstem contains various groups of neurons that are necessary to maintain arousal or wakefulness. In addition, the brainstem controls life-supporting functions, such as breathing and the regulation of blood pressure. In the acute phase, any brain insult can cause a swelling of intracranial tissues, leading to increased pressure, which in turn results in a compression of the brainstem against other structures in the lower portion of the skull (Figure 3.2). In the past, this compression and the temporary impairment of brainstem function had a catastrophic effect—coma, followed by cessation of spontaneous breathing, rapidly leading to cardiac arrest and death.

Figure 3.1 An illustration of the mechanisms of a safety coffin. The drawing is taken from the patent filed on July 4, 1882, by Albert Fearnaught. His particular version was based on the installation of a complicated mechanism, whereby a rope tied around the deceased's wrist, if tugged, would release a spring that, in turn, would open a large colored fan inserted at the upper end of a tube at ground level. The same movement would cause a flap to open and allow fresh air to circulate in the coffin. The patent explains that following interment, the coffin should be frequently checked by the cemetery custodian. It also specifies that the mechanism can be recycled for use in other coffins if the deceased should not return to the world of the living.

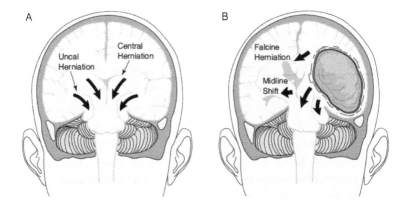

Figure 3.2 A schematic drawing to illustrate the different herniation syndromes seen following increases in intracranial pressure and mass effects. When the volume increase is symmetric in the two hemispheres (A), there may be central herniation, as well as herniation of either or both medial temporal lobes, through the tentorial opening, resulting in brainstem compression. Asymmetric compression (B) may cause herniation of the ipsilateral cingulate gyrus under the falx (falcine herniation). This type of compression may cause distortion of the diencephalon and brainstem by either downward herniation or midline shift.

Today, coma is not necessarily a passage to death. The game changer was the invention of mechanical ventilation. This technique was introduced in clinical practice in 1952 by the Danish doctor Bjorn Ibsen, during the poliomyelitis epidemic of 1952, which in the span of a few weeks, temporarily (but completely) paralyzed hundreds of people, including children [32, 33]. Ibsen inserted tubes into his patients' trachea, which were then connected to a pump, each worked by one of the 200 medical students he had enlisted for the purpose. He organized special wards for this life-supporting activity, so he can also be said to be the inventor of the ICU. His heroic efforts were crowned with success and the mortality rate from poliomyelitis in his area dropped from 90% to just 25%. Mechanical ventilation is, of course, no longer manually operated, the pumps are motorized, and controlled by sensors and computers, which maintain the optimal mix of oxygen and carbon dioxide for months or years if necessary. Today, breathing can be controlled indefinitely and a new chapter has been written in the natural history of coma. In fact, rather unexpectedly, a relatively simple device, such as a pump that inflates the lungs, changed the course of medicine, and moved boundaries that, for ages, where thought to be insuperable and fixed.

First, death has moved from the heart to the brain with important consequences from the clinical, juridical, and anthropological stand points [34]. In the past, death coincided with the cessation of cardiorespiratory functions. A relative was considered dead if a mirror held in front of his lips did not mist over. He had "expired," "drawn his last breath." Then, the doctors could confirm by feeling his pulse and auscultating the heart. The cessation of cardiorespiratory function and the death of the brain were inseparable, the two events were reciprocally linked. Today, mechanical ventilation has broken this vicious circle and cardiorespiratory function can be maintained artificially, with or without a functioning brain. The main result is that many patients can survive the most critical phases of coma, during which brainstem function is temporarily impaired. The other side of the token is that we can encounter the paradox of a body that is still functioning, even if its brain is completely destroyed, liquefied—a moving chest and a beating heart, without a brain. In 1968, a group of 10 doctors, a theologian, a lawyer, and a historian met in Harvard to review the issue. The Harvard Committee, as it was known, had the responsibility of establishing a new criterion with which to define death, which could no longer be cardiorespiratory in nature, but needed to be neurological [35]. The discussion was long and arduous, with doctors becoming lawyers, and the lawyer waxing philosophical, but a decision was finally reached. Death coincides with the irreversible cessation of the functions of the whole brain, brainstem included. From the operational point of view, the process for establishing brain death is complex and requires a number of steps, including verification of complete unresponsiveness; the cessation of all functions and reflexes of the brainstem, spontaneous breathing included; and (depending on the specific legislation of the country) the instrumental documentation of the absence of electrical and metabolic activity in the brain. In point of fact, brain death identifies a particular, artificial situation where, to all extents and purposes, the body is decapitated (the nervous system above the spinal cord is completely destroyed), but continues to receive oxygen through external machines. Death decreed, based on neurological criteria, may be even harder for the patient's nearest to accept, as his outward appearance is often healthy, the chest rising, the skin warm and rosy. Today, this delicate task lies with the doctor. On the other hand, a diagnosis of brain death is necessarily more accurate than that established by the cessation of the respiratory and circulatory functions, even if it is less intuitive. The new frontier of death is very clear, and does not admit any possibility of error or recovery.

While the introduction of the mechanical ventilator has helped to establish a new clear divide between life and death, it has played havoc with the borders of consciousness [36, 37]. Millions of patients with devastating cerebral lesions, which only 50 years ago would have been lethal, now survive the comatose state and may slip into medical conditions that were previously unknown. In fact, following a coma there is now a range of possible states—between brain death and conscious awakening—which at present can only be classified in provisional terms.

A patient who survives coma will typically start opening his eyes after 2 weeks or so. This is the sign that the coma is coming to an end. The patient's eyes open because the brainstem starts to function again, so guaranteeing spontaneous respiration and the recovery of what the neurologists call vigilance, but is commonly known as wakefulness. The part of the brainstem that is closest to the spinal cord (the so-called "medulla oblongata") is primarily involved in the maintenance of the functioning of the cardiorespiratory systems, while the upper parts, the pons and the midbrain, house extremely important neurons, called the activating system, which control eyes opening and establish whether the brain is generally switched off or on, in a state of sleep or wakefulness [31]. When these neurons fire-up in a healthy brain (which happens every morning upon awakening), the muscular tone increases, the eyes open and the person regains awareness of the self and the surrounding world. In a brain that has suffered severe damage, this does not necessarily happen. Brainstem neurons may activate, spontaneous breathing recovers, and the eyes open, but this does not mean that consciousness returns [30, 38]. It is like flicking a switch when the bulb has burnt out. A click, with no light. In fact, the recovery of brainstem functions, although necessary, is not, in itself, sufficient for awakening to be accompanied by the recovery of subjective experience.

Some patients open their eyes, breathe spontaneously, and appear to be awake, but do not show voluntary behavior, do not respond to simple orders, and do not react purposely to painful stimuli. This condition of unresponsive wakefulness was originally defined by Bryan Jannet and Fred Plum in 1972 as the vegetative state (VS) [39], a diagnostic term that is now been replaced by the more descriptive and neutral label unresponsive wakefulness syndrome (UWS) [40]. This is a strange situation as we are used to associating eye-opening with the recovery of consciousness; after all, this is what happens every morning when we arise out of our nightly oblivion. Hence, we naturally tend to interpret the open position of the eyelid as a master power-on indicator, as the sign that consciousness is turned on. In this man-made condition, however, brought about as it is by medical technology, this intuition is wrong—eyelids and orbs are just things moved by the primitive, blind force of the brainstem. In these patients, there is often an increase in muscle tone and a range of automatic gestures, but these are unintentional and without meaning—the eyes move without pursuing a target, there are reflex movements of the limbs and neck, grimaces, chewing movements, utterances, and sometimes uncontrolled outbursts of laughter and tears. The vegetative state/unresponsive wakefulness syndrome (VS/UWS) obviously differs from the internal decapitation of brain death and it differs from coma in that the patient is awake. The only thing missing, or at least, all that appears to be missing judging by behavior, is that spark of consciousness.

However, the VS/UWS is just one of the new offspring of coma. Some patients may come out of a coma, open their eyes, recover self-awareness, and recognize the world around them, but remain totally paralyzed. Unfortunately, this is not the temporary paralysis of anesthesia awareness, but a permanent state caused by neuronal damage. Such paralyses are often caused by a very small lesion (maybe only a few centimeters in extension), but they are, nonetheless, devastating because it affects a key spot in the brainstem where all the fibers (and there are hundreds of thousands), which carry motor commands from the cerebral cortex to the spinal cord, meet and proceed in a single "bundle." The resulting condition is known as "locked-in syndrome" (LIS) [30, 41], which is a poignant rendering of the sense of isolation that characterizes this state. It is not uncommon for LIS patients to be diagnosed as VS/UWS, particularly during the first few months of disease [42].

Fortunately, in time, most of these patients recover the control of some extrinsic eye muscles, and become able to shift their gaze up and down, or blink. These movements are governed by motor fibers that leave the brainstem before the area of the lesion. In some cases, it is the patients' relatives who realize that these eye movements are not random automatic patterns, but represent a desperate and laborious attempt to communicate consciousness. Once they have been identified as LIS, these patients learn to use eye movements to establish a binary code and initiate a communication process, which at the beginning is very basic (yes/no), but can become progressively more efficient as time passes. Using this fragile output channel, literally reduced to a single thread that connects the cerebral cortex to the muscles of the eye, LIS patients can finally write and communicate their conscious universe, as well as hunger, thirst, pain, desperation, happiness [43–45]. Many LIS patients who do manage to communicate with the external world, report that their quality of life is not very much different to that reported by healthy controls [46]. This rather surprising finding is very revealing. It suggests, on the one hand, that healthy subjects tend to complain too much about their own existence. On the other, it shows that a locked-in brain can access an internal universe that is large and interesting enough to replace the one that cannot be actively explored. Of course, this all depends on the patients' conscious existence being acknowledged and on an adequate level of support. Unfortunately, there are patients in which not even eye movements are preserved. This rare condition, where all outputs are blocked, is known as "complete locked-in syndrome" [47]. In this case, the anguish and the sense of impotence described by the anesthesiologist who regained awareness in a fully paralyzed body may become a permanent state. The possibility of even a single human being in such a condition of incommunicable existence is a fact that is hard to accept.

There are no limits to variety in the outcomes of intensive care medicine; in fact, there are a plethora of conditions between LIS and VS/UWS, which have been classified collectively as a "minimally conscious state" (MCS). MCS was only officially recognized as distinct from the VS/UWS in 2002 [36], which testifies to our still provisional understanding of what may happen after a coma and provides an inkling of the changes that we can expect over the coming decades [48]. Patients who are unable communicate their thoughts and feelings, but occasionally show inconsistent, but discernible signs of consciousness, are considered as being in a MCS. A classic example is the brain-injured subject who, in a context of general unresponsiveness, occasionally appears to track, with purposeful eye movements, doctors and relatives as they move about the room.

These minimal signs of consciousness change from one day to another, from one minute to the next, and are difficult to extrapolate from a background of intense automatic activity. For example, it is very difficult to decide whether a finger twitch or the bats of an eyelid are involuntary reflexes or voluntary attempts to interact with the environment. It is equally difficult to judge whether an eruption of laughter or suddenly bursting into tears reflects a conscious emotional content or just the mechanical consequence of the random discharge of a small group of neurons surviving in the depth of the brain. Therefore, the diagnosis of MCS can only be reached through a careful, detailed, and repeated evaluation of the patient's behavior. Accurate detection of MCS patients is extremely important, as these patients retain some form of experience, even though we do not know to what extent or of what. Probably, this state covers a multitude of conditions that we will never know or understand because they cannot be communicated. It is possible that some patients may only have a fragmented glimmer of consciousness, rather similar to what healthy individuals experience as they sink into slumber, others may fluctuate in a sort of dream world or delirium, while others still may be completely lucid and conscious, but without any reliable means of communicating this. There is another reason why an accurate diagnosis is important: unlike patients in a VS/UWS, MCS patients have a better chance of recovery even after years of illness [49, 50], particularly if they undergo intensive rehabilitation programs.

Unfortunately, detecting consciousness in patients who are unable to communicate remains difficult, and MCS patients are a paradigmatic example of this problem. Recent data show that nearly half of the patient labelled as being in an unconscious VS/UWS are actually in a MCS [51–53]; this low sensitivity in detecting conscious existence represents one of the most serious clinical and ethical issues of contemporary neurology. According to a rough estimate, in the United States alone, there are 280,000 MCS patients, the equivalent of the population of a major city [54]. How many more are not recognized and end up dying in places with lower standards of care? How can consciousness escape our radar so easily? To better understand the reasons behind this diagnostic error, let us step into the shoes of a detective in search of signs of conscious experience.

Level 1: Sensory Inputs and Motor Outputs

Classically, the decision as to whether a patient is conscious or not is made based on a stimulus–response paradigm. This is the first, fundamental level of investigation. Since the physical mechanisms of subjective experience are unknown, we treat the brain as a black box and assess consciousness based on input–output relationships (Figure 3.3A).

A series of standardized tests using verbal and sensory stimuli (visual, acoustic, tactile, and pain) have been established for this purpose; scores are attributed based on the responses given and the spontaneous behavior observed. In very general terms, this clinical approach is not so different from the Turing test. The underlying principle is that the more specific, reproducible, and articulated the responses are, the higher the level of consciousness is. A patient who is able to open his mouth, clench his right fist, left fist, open his eyes, and smile when requested to do so, will be given a higher score than a patient who in response to all these commands only opens his mouth. The most effective of these scales is the coma recovery scale—revised (CRS-R), specifically designed to recognize the faint signs that characterize the passage from the VS/UWS to the MCS [55]. This scale represents the gold standard and its repeated, careful administration is the cornerstone of an accurate assessment of behavioral consciousness. If a patient shows purposeful motor activity, and responds to stimuli in a way that is specific and reproducible, there is no doubt that he is conscious.

On the other hand, even the CRS-R is not watertight [56]. As was mentioned earlier, a dissociation between experience and motor outputs can happen during anesthesia awareness due to NBDs. A fortiori, motor responses may be blocked at multiple levels in neurological syndromes. For example, in amyotrophic lateral sclerosis [57] or in some disorders of the peripheral nerves, such as the Guillain–Barré syndrome [58], the generation and conduction of electrical impulses from the motor cortex to the muscles may be severely impeded. Often, ischemic, hemorrhagic or traumatic lesions may interrupt or tear off the bundles of fibers that

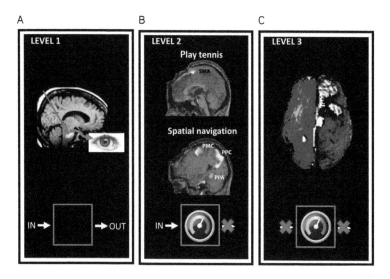

Figure 3.3 The different levels at which consciousness can be assessed. (A) Level 1: when sensory processing (IN, input) and motor behavior (OUT, output) are preserved, the behavioral evaluation can be effective in detecting consciousness, even in the extreme case of locked-in patients. In these patients, a pontine lesion (such as the one indicated by the red arrow) spares the motor nerve controlling vertical eye movements and blinking, through which an effective communication system can be implemented. (B) Level 2: when motor outputs are completely blocked (red cross), but sensory processing is preserved, active fMRI paradigms, in which neuronal responses to verbal instructions are recorded directly from the cerebral cortex can be used. In this example an otherwise unresponsive patient produces specific neuronal activations in response to verbal instructions, such as "imagine you are playing tennis" (top) or "imagine you are walking through your home" (bottom). (C) Level 3: when both sensory processing and motor behavior are impaired, such as in the case of disconnected cortical islands that show preserved activity levels (as indicated here by high PET activity in the right hemisphere), assessing consciousness requires opening the black-box of the brain and identifying the full neural correlates of consciousness.

run from the cerebral cortex to the spinal cord [47]. At a higher level, the basal ganglia and/or the frontal areas of the cerebral cortex may be destroyed or disabled, leading to a loss of motor initiative [59–61]. In all these cases, consciousness can be present, but voluntary motor activity is impeded. So, while a specific, purposeful response can be taken as the definite evidence of the presence of consciousness, the absence of such movements in a brain-damaged patient cannot exclude it. Put simply, the absence of the proof (no motor behavior) cannot be said to be proof of the absence (no conscious experience), and further investigation is required to solve the case.

Level 2: Sensory Inputs and Neural Outputs

At this point, the consciousness detective needs to dig deeper in order to identify those patients who are willing to respond to commands, but cannot because of motor impairment. Ideally, one should be able to detect the neural reflections of a patient's intentions directly, before the electrical impulses that carry the actual motor command are blocked on their way down to the muscles (Figure 3.3B). Incredible as it sounds, this is now possible, as demonstrated by an emblematic case that attracted much attention in scientific circles and beyond. The story began like the story of many other patients; a young girl in her twenties was involved in a serious road accident and suffered a devastating brain trauma. When she was admitted to the emergency room, a computed tomography (CT) scan showed a cerebral hemorrhage and extensive lesions to the frontal cerebral cortex. As often happens after a trauma, the brain swelled, thus increasing pressure inside the cranium. For this reason, the brain stem was squeezed downwards against the rigid structures at the base of the cranium and the patient entered a state of coma. To prevent irreversible brainstem damage (potentially leading to brain death), the neurosurgeons removed a part of the skull to alleviate the internal pressure and, after a few days, the patient opened her eyes spontaneously and emerged from coma. Bedside behavioral tests revealed only reflex activity; the eyes were open, but did not fixate nor track, the head did not turn toward stimuli, arms and legs showed no purposeful movements. The tests were repeated after a few months with the same outcome—no voluntary movement, no response to stimuli, no sign of awareness of the self or the surrounding environment. The patient was awake, but appeared to be unconscious and the criteria for the diagnosis of a VS/UWS were met. That is, until a team of neuroscientists from the University of Cambridge and the University of Liege decided to run a very important test.

The team had just completed a study on a group of healthy individuals demonstrating that it is possible to "read" a person's intentions directly from brain activity [62]. The readings were very coarse, but reliable. The participants were given a functional magnetic resonance imaging (fMRI) scan, which estimated the variations in the amount of oxygen consumed by neurons. The greater the number of impulses generated by the neurons, the more oxygen they consumed, so when the variations were processed by a computer, they provide the input for detailed maps of brain activity. The scientists discovered that, when a healthy volunteer was asked to imagine that they were playing tennis, specific parts of the frontal cerebral cortex (the supplementary motor area), which are involved in planning movement, are clearly activated; however, when the same person was asked to imagine navigating through his own apartment (say, from the bedroom to the kitchen), a very different constellation of brain areas (including the posterior parietal lobe, the parahippocampal gyrus deep in the core of the brain, and the lateral premotor cortex), involved in the processing of spatial coordinates and the memory of places, lit up. Looking at the neural activation maps on the monitor, the Cambridge–Liege research team were able to say, with a high degree of accuracy, whether the person (who was lying motionless in the scanner) was actually thinking of playing tennis or of walking through her apartment. Hence, by employing this protocol, called active paradigm, an external observer can judge whether a subject is willfully responding to specific instructions completely independent of motor behavior.

Encouraged by their success with healthy individuals, the team, led by Adrian Owen and Steven Laureys, decided to assess the efficacy of the technique on the young patient who had been diagnosed as being in VS/UWS. Undaunted by her lack of response and immobility, the scientists painstakingly explained the experiment; she was told that, at a certain point, in time she would be asked to imagine doing certain things and that she should then concentrate on mentally engaging in these activities. They then pushed her bed into the narrow tunnel of the fMRI scanner. After a few minutes the scanner started to detect the metabolic reflections of neural activity, and the researcher in the control room issued his instructions using a microphone connected to headphones. When the girl was asked to imagine playing tennis, her muscles remained still, but neurons in the supplementary motor cortex started to become active; the anterior region of the brain lit up bright red, showing a significant increase in oxygen consumption. Just a coincidence? Shortly after, the researcher told her to imagine navigating through her home, and neural activity split and shifted to a different set of brain regions, just as in the healthy subjects. The test was repeated several times, and the results were consistent. The patient was present, understood the instructions, wanted to respond and did so with her neurons. Shortly after, in September 2006, the results of the experiment were published in the prestigious scientific magazine *Science* [63], confirming what until then had just been an unsettling doubt. There are conscious brains that can actually escape the behavioral radar. This finding marked the beginning of an astonishing scientific adventure, with profound implications that can be fully appreciated through the words of Adrian Owen himself [64].[1] How many patients are lying in hospital wards and nursing homes, in a state on non-behavioral consciousness? What do they think? What do they want? After this first breakthrough, the Cambridge–Liege team extended the experiment to a number of other cases, and were able to demonstrate that the first was not an isolated incident (see also [65]). Then, they showed even more—a few VS/UWS patients can even establish a slow, rudimentary form of communication, through which they can answer simple questions—imagine to play tennis to say "yes," spatial navigation to say "no" [66]. The finding represents a milestone with profound ethical and legal implication (see, for example, [67], [37] and [68]) that we will not explore in this context. Here, let us go back to the problem of reliably detecting consciousness.

Can we use brain responses to verbal commands to solve the problem once and for all? Unfortunately, not. As the Cambridge–Liege researchers point out, there are too many brain-injured patients (over 80%) who are conscious, as judged by the usual behavioral standards, but are unable to voluntarily activate specific neurons in a brain scan

---

1 In this engaging and moving book the author tells the story of his journey in search for communication with patients lost in the grey zone at the outer boundary of consciousness.

[66]. That is, there are too many "false negatives," meaning that the "imagine playing tennis" fMRI test has a low sensitivity. The problem is that, although following the instructions to imagine playing tennis is fairly simple for healthy individuals, the same task can be far too challenging for a person who has suffered brain damage [69]. There are, in fact, numerous reasons for this: in the first place, many brain-damaged patients are aphasic, they are no longer able to understand verbal language and, therefore, the instructions mean nothing to them. Others do not have the necessary reserves of concentration and attention. Other patients may have suffered lesions to the very regions of the brain that are necessary to imagine playing tennis or navigating through the environment. Then, there are those who are simply too depressed, demotivated, confused, to want to participate in what might appear to be a senseless game, requiring an extra active effort they are reluctant to make. To make things more complicated, recording neural activity with fMRI in non-collaborating patients is extremely challenging, as even slight uncontrolled head movements may confound data interpretation. At this point, the consciousness detective has to come to terms with the fact that, even in the case of the fMRI active paradigm, the absence of proof is not proof of absence.

Of course, researchers and clinicians have tried other methods that require less effort on the patient's part and present less technical challenges. One example is the P3, an electrical response to sensory stimuli that can be registered by sticking a few electroencephalogram (EEG) electrodes on the patient's scalp. This EEG response was first described 50 years ago [70] and was called P3 because it had a positive polarity and because it occurs roughly 300 ms after the onset of a sensory stimulus A good way to elicit this response is by presenting a less frequent "target" or "oddball" stimulus together with more frequent "standard" stimuli, such as when a high-pitch tone ("beep") is embedded in a sequence of lower-pitch stimuli ("boop"). A P3-like wave can also be elicited by administering "oddball" sequences of stimuli ("boop, boop, boop, boop, boop") amongst a series of more frequent standard sequences ("boop, boop, boop, boop, beep") [71]. In all cases, the necessary condition for the P3 wave to occur is that the "oddball" sensory event needs to be related to the task at hand in some way; for example, the subject must be instructed to pay attention, and count the infrequent events or to react to them overtly with a button press. Thus, in healthy volunteers the P3 component is present only when the individual is attentive and aware of the rule. If a subject forgets the rules, becomes distracted by another task, or starts mind-wandering, the P3 vanishes [72]. In other words, the presence of this late EEG response suggests that the subject has received, attended, detected, and actively manipulated in her mind a specific sensory event. Importantly, a P3 can be found in some unresponsive patients [73], confirming the possibility that conscious sensory processing can be preserved, even in the absence of motor behavior. Thus, the P3 has recently been proposed as a signature of consciousness and as a test to be applied at the bedside of brain-injured patients [74, 75]. Is the P3 sensitive enough to serve as a dependable consciousness screening? When one examines the performance of this test in the case of MCS patients, a P3b is present in only 14% of the cases [73, 76]. So, similarly to the fMRI active paradigm, the P3 can reveal the presence of covert consciousness in particular patients, but generally suffers from low sensitivity. Practically, if a detective was to search for signs of awareness in the ICU or in a rehabilitation center using the P3 as a test, he would miss eight conscious patients out of 10. The reason for this does not rest in a technical detail (the method is extremely simple), but in a general confound; it is becoming now clear that this late brain response does not reflect conscious perception, as such, but rather cognitive processes that follow conscious perception such as working memory, executive functions, task planning and reporting [77–79]. Recent paradigms, called no-report paradigms, during which participants become aware of a particular sensory event, but are not requested to actively report their percept, show that conscious experience can occur without a P3 [80]. Likewise, the P3 can be absent in a heathy subject who is blissfully aware of the light shimmering on the waves at sunset, as well as in a brain-injured patient who is immersed in his own memories, in a vivid hallucination, or worse, in excruciating pain.

Finally, there is a more fundamental problem for approaches based on the administration of sensory stimuli or commands, however: consciousness may be present with or without sensory processing. We all know this because it happens almost every night, when we dream. During dreaming complex, temporally unfolding hallucinatory episodes can be as intense and vivid as waking experiences—yet sensory stimuli are ignored to the point that they are rarely incorporated into experience [81, 82]. Consciousness may also completely disconnect from the external environment during some forms of anesthesia. Some dissociative esthetic agents, such as ketamine at high doses, are known to induce a dream-like hallucinatory state associated with sensory disconnection and complete unresponsiveness [83]. Similar disconnections and dissociations may occur in pathological conditions, whereby many patients may be conscious, but fail to produce the right neuronal responses to external stimuli just because their sensory pathways and cortices are disconnected or functionally disabled. Other patients may just be somewhere else, in states that are not easily accessible. It is difficult to understand how it feels to be in such a condition, just as it is hard to imagine how it feels to perceive the world through the echolocation of a bat.

> [...] There was something and the *something* was not nothing. The nearest label for the something might possibly be "awareness", but that could be misleading, since any awareness I'd ever had before the accident was *my* awareness, my awareness of one thing or another. In contrast, this *something*, if it be called awareness, had no *I* as its *subject* and no content as its object. It just was.

This is the first-person account of the aftermath of a mild traumatic brain injury from which the subject recovered promptly [84]. Notably, even subtler alterations of neuronal functioning may lead to unusual states. Consider, for example, how it feels to recover from syncope [85]:

> [...] at the beginning of coming to, one has a certain moment of vague, limitless infinite feeling—a sense of *existence in general* without the least trace of distinction between the me and not-me

These descriptions of disconnected, unbound experience are relevant for two reasons. First, because they underscore, once more, a fundamental notion—consciousness can exist—in and of itself—as a state of pure presence devoid of any perceptual object, self-monitoring or acting, during which input and output are not necessary and no function is performed. Second, these accidental reports give a rough idea of the alien experiences that patients stricken by more severe brain injuries may have, without being able to tell. The fact of the matter is that intensive care medicine is artificially producing, as a by-product of saving many lives, new kinds of brains that may remain isolated, split, or fragmented; in the extreme case, large cortical islands, or an archipelago of islands, may survive that are totally disconnected from the world outside [86]. Can these islands maintain a capacity for some form of experience? That is, does it feel like anything to be a big chunk of isolated human cortex? For now, we cannot answer the question. What we know is that, in such cases, assessing consciousness based on inputs and outputs would be ineffective.

Level 3: Into the Black Box

If we do not want to miss anyone out, we clearly need to find ways to assess consciousness independent of sensory processing and motor behavior; this is the last resort, which requires opening the black box of the brain (Figure 3.3C). The problem basically boils down to addressing the instinctive question bugging the student struck by the cerebrum on his palm. What is special about a conscious piece of matter? There must be a difference that makes a difference in the inner workings of the brain! Something that is always there when consciousness is present, something measurable that goes away when the brain ceases to host a subject and becomes a dull object. Only that now, having considered the possibility of conscious cortical islands, the existential and philosophical flavor of the problem leaves space to the bitter taste of the urgent ethical question.

In 1907 Douncan McDougall, put six men on a precision commercial scale and found a difference of 21 g at the moment of their dying. Before Dr McDougall could publish his results, the *New York Times* broke the story with an article entitled "Soul as weight, physician, thinks" (Figure 3.4). The finding was finally published in *Journal of the American Society for Psychical Research*, only to be disproved soon after because of fundamental methodological flaws and lack of experimental control.

Today, we have far better scales and shared methodological standards, yet, weighing consciousness directly in the brain remains a challenging task. Like astronomers, we must be ready to capture the faintest of signals, movements of waves and particles, far reflections of a star that cannot be observed with the naked eye. Yet it is still quite easy to blunder.

Scientifically, the challenge boils down to identifying the neural mechanisms that are necessary and sufficient for being conscious in a

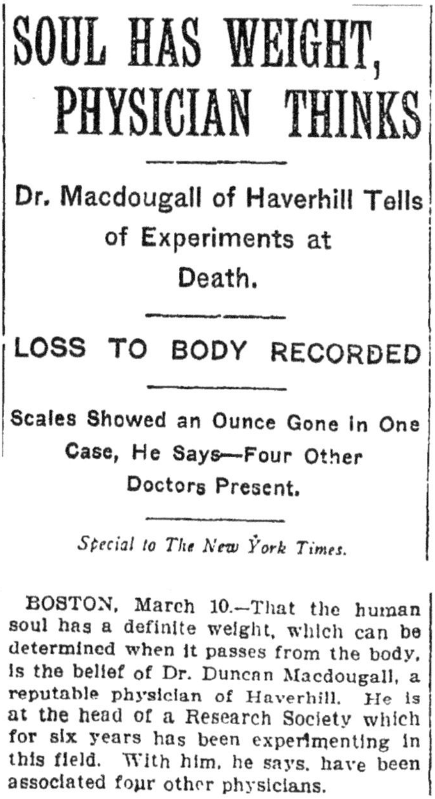

SOUL HAS WEIGHT, PHYSICIAN THINKS

Dr. Macdougall of Haverhill Tells
of Experiments at
Death.

LOSS TO BODY RECORDED

Scales Showed an Ounce Gone in One
Case, He Says—Four Other
Doctors Present.

Special to The New York Times.

BOSTON, March 10.—That the human soul has a definite weight, which can be determined when it passes from the body, is the belief of Dr. Duncan Macdougall, a reputable physician of Haverhill. He is at the head of a Research Society which for six years has been experimenting in this field. With him, he says, have been associated four other physicians.

Figure 3.4 The *New York Times* article reporting Douncan McDougall's findings in 1907.

broad sense. We think it is important to reaffirm once again that what we are looking for here is very different from the neuronal correlates of a specific conscious content (say a face, a sound, or an imaginary task). Here, we are dealing with a more fundamental quest, the one for the neural correlates of a general capacity for any form of conscious experience, otherwise called the full neural correlates of consciousness [87]. Empirically, the task involves screening different features of neural activity to identify the brain-based index that yields the best accuracy; that is, a measure that ideally has maximum specificity (it is always low when consciousness is absent) and maximum sensitivity (it is always high when any form of consciousness is present). Can such an index be found? To address this question, it is helpful to go through a quick overview of the different aspects of brain activity that have been considered so far as possible full neuronal correlates of consciousness.

Global Activity Levels

Let's start with the obvious candidate. The first idea that springs to mind is that plainly measuring overall levels of brain activity may represent a viable strategy. Maybe consciousness is most intense when the brain is most active and fades when it shuts down—as simple as that. We know that the cranium is crammed full of neurons and that each of these can emit a variable number of electrical impulses (from 0 to 400) every second. One could thus start from the basic hypothesis that consciousness is related to the quantity of electrical impulses; if this were true, it would greatly simplify matters—a recording made with any one of the available techniques to gauge global levels of neuronal activity [fMRI, positron-emission tomography (PET)] would do, even in the case of a totally unresponsive patient. A subject whose neurons engage in frenetic neural activity would be more conscious that one with just some groups of neurons buzzing here and there, and a patient with no active neurons would be unconscious. There is, in fact, a coarse relationship between overall activity levels and the brain's capacity for consciousness, if only because preserved levels of brain activity indicate that neurons and their basic metabolic capabilities are still in functioning order. However, this relationship is far from direct and there are many exceptions. For example, intracerebral recordings show that, during the deepest stages of non-rapid eye movement (NREM) sleep, when consciousness fades almost completely, average firing rates of cortical neurons can be as high, if not higher, than during wakefulness [88, 89]. Epileptic seizures provide another striking example; during many generalized seizures, consciousness is lost, yet the brain is super-active, with neurons firing as intensely as they can (Figure 3.5A) [90]! The brain activity = consciousness equation is also challenged by the findings of studies on brain-damaged patients. While it is true that patients who are comatose or VS/UWS usually show a decrease in cerebral metabolism and that preserved metabolism is a good prognostic marker of future recovery [91], it is also true that global activity rates do not necessarily increase when patients recover consciousness [92]. The truth of the matter is that consciousness can disappear even when the level of neural activity is normal (or even higher than normal), and can reappear when brain metabolism is much reduced. In short, a simple count of overall brain activity levels does not provide a valid consciousness meter.

Activity in Specific Regions of the Brain.

An alternative possibility is that activity in some privileged brain regions may be crucial for consciousness. For example, the frontal lobe has been traditionally thought to be in a special position because of its evolutionary profile, and its role in decision-making and self-reflection. After all, many think that the frontal lobe is what makes us human and we know that we are a conscious species. Over the past two decades, several experiments have been performed comparing brain responses to sensory stimuli that are or are not consciously perceived, as indicated by the subject's report [74]. The results of these experiments suggest that, when a subject reports that he/she has seen a stimulus, there is a sudden "ignition" of a wave of neuronal activity, which reverberates between the back of the brain to the frontal cortex. This frontoparietal activation has been proposed as a general signature of consciousness. Is this frontal ignition the difference that makes the difference between unconsciousness and consciousness? If this were the case, one could aim an activity meter directly to the frontal cortex, in order to reliably read out a subject's state of consciousness. This idea is appealing in its intuitive simplicity, but seems less plausible if one ponders its rationale and the data carefully. First, the design of the experiments highlighting the role of the frontal lobe essentially rely on the subjects' capacity to decide whether they saw or heard something, and their willingness to communicate their decision. In fact, the explosive activation of the frontal lobe, just like the P3 described earlier, tends to fade when the subjects still consciously perceive the stimulus, but are not asked to report on it [93, 94]. Second, the view that the anterior part of the brain is necessary for the generation of subjective experience must confront the evidence obtained from lesion studies that consciousness can be present, even after massive frontal lesions. For example, complete bilateral frontal lobectomy and large bilateral prefrontal resections, once performed in some psychiatric patients, do not impair consciousness [95]. Likewise, prefrontal lobotomy and leucotomy, in which the prefrontal cortex is cut off from its thalamic inputs, do not impair consciousness [96]. Notably, neurological

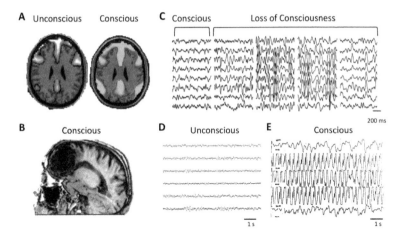

A Unconscious   Conscious   **C** Conscious   Loss of Consciousness

200 ms

B Conscious

D Unconscious   **E** Conscious

1 s   1 s

Figure 3.5 The empirical search for full neural correlates of consciousness: problems and exceptions. (A) Voxel-by-voxel maps of the mean percentage change in fMRI signals during absence seizures: large-scale frontoparietal activity increases during the loss of consciousness (warm colors) and decreases during recovery of consciousness (cool colors). (B) A young man who had fallen on an iron spike that completely penetrated both of his frontal lobes causing an extensive bilateral lesion affecting orbital, dorsolateral, and mesial regions of the prefrontal cortex, who nevertheless, went on to live a stable family life—marrying and raising two children— in an appropriate professional and social setting. Although displaying many of the typical frontal lobe behavioral disturbances, he never complained of loss of sensory perception nor did he show visual or other deficits. (C) Spontaneous EEG activity showing the emergence of hypersynchronous alpha (10–12 Hz) rhythms during loss of consciousness induced by propofol anesthesia. (D) Low-amplitude alpha rhythms can be recorded in unconscious patients in severe post-anoxic coma. (E) Conversely, high-amplitude bilateral slow waves may be observed in awake, conscious patients, during some form of non-convulsive status epilepticus.

Figure 3.5 (Panel A) Reprinted from *Consciousness and Cognition*, 35 N. Noy, S. Bickel, E. Zion-Golumbic, M. Harel, T. Golan, I. Davidesco, C. A. Schevon, G. M. McKhann, R. R. Goodman, C. E. Schroeder, A. D. Mehta, and R. Malach, Ignition's glow: ultra-fast spread of global cortical activity accompanying local "ignitions" in visual cortex during conscious visual perception, pp. 206–24, https://doi.org/10.1016/j.concog.2015.03.006. Copyright © 2015, with permission from Elsevier Inc. (Panel B) Adapted with permission from *JAMA Neurology*, 58 (7) Mataró, M., Jurado, M.A., García-Sánchez, C. *et al*. Long-term effects of bilateral frontal brain lesion: 60 years after injury with an iron bar, pp. 1139–42, Figure 3c, doi:10.1001/archneur.58.7.1139. Copyright © 2001, American Medical Association, with permission. All rights reserved. (Panel C) Reprinted from *Current Biology*, 23(6), Gernot G. Supp, Markus Siegel, Joerg F. Hipp, and Andreas K. Engel, Cortical hypersynchrony predicts breakdown of sensory processing during loss of consciousness, pp. 1988–93, https://doi.org/10.1016/j.cub.2011.10.017. © 2011 Elsevier Ltd., with permission from Elsevier Ltd. (Panel D) Reproduced with permission from *Journal of the* patients with extensive bilateral prefrontal damage (Figure 3.5B) may have grossly deficient scores in tests of frontal lobe function, but intact perceptual abilities, and are obviously conscious and, indeed, conduct a nearly normal life [97–99]. Taken together, the data suggest that frontal portions of the cortical network may play a prominent role in reflection, working memory, reporting and in the control and execution of many cognitive tasks, but are not necessary for consciousness [87, 100]. In essence, the anterior part of the brain seems to be more concerned with doing, rather than with being. In fact, the strongest correlation between activity and absence/presence of experience in both physiological [101] and pathological conditions [102] is found in the posteromedial cortex. This correlation is statistically significant at the group-level and points to the existence of a posterior hot zone for consciousness, but it is still far from providing a reliable index to assess consciousness objectively in individual subjects.

Levels of Neuronal Synchrony

Maybe measuring global or regional levels of neuronal activity is not enough; maybe what really matters is not so much the quantity of neuronal activity, but its quality. In recent years, much attention has been dedicated to the phenomenon of synchronization, the ability of neural groups distributed across distant brain regions to fire their impulses in a coordinated fashion. Synchronization can be measured by simultaneously recording the activations produced by various areas of the brain and by computing their relative timing. The EEG is the ideal instrument for this type of assessment because it can detect neuronal activity with great precision, down to milliseconds; thus, when distant groups of neurons fire together (say, within the same 20–30 ms window), the EEG oscillations recorded by the various electrodes show a high temporal correlation and are defined as "synchronized." The idea that there is a connection between the synchronization of neural impulses and consciousness derives from the observation that, in many experimental conditions, the conscious perception of a complex object, such as a face, is typically accompanied by rapid bursts (30–70 Hz) of electrical activity that is correlated across distant regions of the brain [103–105]. This experimental evidence ties in well with the reasonable assumption that consciousness requires "binding" together a multitude of attributes within a single experience [106]. Hence, transient synchronization may be the mechanisms by which distant groups of neurons that process different sensory features (vertical and horizontal lines, colors, and movements) come together when a subject recognizes a complex object, such as a face. This empirical evidence led to the hypothesis that synchronization, above and beyond levels of activations, may be the essential mechanism of consciousness. Hence, over the last two decades, a large number of experiments have been performed where the degree of temporal correlation between EEG oscillations was studied in various conditions, in which consciousness comes and go, including wakefulness, sleep, epilepsy, and disorders of consciousness. Is there a straightforward relationship between the degree of large-scale neuronal synchronization and the capacity for consciousness? Although measures of temporal correlation provide interesting results at the group level [107, 108], there are too many exceptions to the rule. Indeed, synchronization does not necessarily decrease when consciousness fades and there are various conditions in which neuronal activity can even become hyper-synchronous when consciousness is lost. For example, neuronal synchrony can be preserved during NREM sleep [88], and even enhanced following the administration of many anesthetic agents that induce loss of consciousness [109] (Figure 3.5C). Crucially, during generalized seizures, billions of neurons across the whole cortical mantle start firing in tight synchrony, which should result in maximal binding, but consciousness vanishes, rather than becoming more vivid [110, 111]. Overall, there seems to be some kind of balance—there must be some degree of synchrony for conscious experience to be there, but not too much of it, otherwise consciousness fades. Yet, we do not have a clear theoretical rationale for this, neither we have a useful decisional cut-off based on the optimal synchrony level that we could use to detect consciousness in individual patients.

Slow Waves and Fast Rhythms

In spite of the recent attempts to squeeze out quantitative indices of consciousness using sophisticated algorithms, the simple observation of the EEG trace may still represent one of the most sensitive and useful marker available. The notion of a basic relationship between the shape of brain waves and the level of consciousness is a legacy of Hans Berger, the pioneer of human EEG. Almost 100 years ago, Berger noticed that subjects who were fully alert and responsive showed low-voltage, fast waves (more than 8/s), which became progressively larger and slower as they became drowsy and fell asleep [112]. This general correlation has been duly confirmed over the following decades [113, 114]. Now, we know well that high-voltage slow waves tend to be prominent during NREM sleep early in the night when subjects, if awakened, often claim they were not conscious at all [115]. Likewise, a sudden increase in slow waves coincides with the behavioral loss of consciousness upon induction of general anesthesia [116, 117]. In a clinical context, the changing pattern of waves from large, slow waves to low-frequency faster EEG oscillations correlates at the group level with the progression from the VS/UWS, to the MCS, to behavioral consciousness [118]. Nevertheless, distinguishing conscious from unconscious individuals simply based on the amplitude and the frequency of scalp EEG oscillations is not always reliable, as a significant overlap exists between VS/UWS and MCS patients [76, 119]. Again, when it comes to single cases, there are many exceptions. For example, some unconscious patients who are in a severe post-anoxic coma show steady, widespread fast (10 Hz) rhythm, rather than slow waves [120] (Figure 3.5D) Conversely, in some cases consciousness is present but there are large slow waves, as after the administration of atropine [121, 122] or in some forms of status epilepticus [123, 124] (Figure 3.5E). An interesting possibility is that, in such patients, slow wave activity may only involve some cortical areas, but not others. Indeed, intracranial electrical recordings show that, during sleep, some cortical areas may become activated, while the scalp EEG is still dominated by slow waves [125] and source modeling reveals that such locally activated EEG over a parieto-occipital region just before awakening from slow-wave sleep occurs when participants report visual dreams, even though other cortical areas display low-frequency activity at this time [101]. Thus, it may be that local, rather than global, cortical activation is important for consciousness, but these aspects are difficult to assess reliably based on the spontaneous scalp EEG alone.

So, our investigation ends here for the time being. To detect consciousness reliably in another human being, under all circumstances, is much more difficult than it seems, and the methods and instruments that are currently available are not yet equal to the task. Observing behavioral outputs to sensory stimuli is not enough because patients may be unable to move. Directly detecting neuronal activations in response to commands or sensory inputs may overcome motor blockage, but lacks sensitivity because patients may be conscious, but disconnected from the external environment, distracted, or not interested in performing the requested task. Even when we try to go beyond input–output relationships by directly peeking into the black box of the brain using advanced tools, we cannot unequivocally solve this issue. We may obtain significant average effects at the population level in some conditions, but lower accuracy when it comes to individual subjects across different conditions. This is particularly frustrating considering the triumphs, real or apparent, that technical developments have supported in other fields of brain research. Every year scientific articles and commentaries in the general press report spectacular breakthroughs, leading us to believe that the relation between mind and brain no longer holds any secrets. The cerebral areas of empathy have been tracked down and identified, as have those areas that seem to make the difference between being truly in love and faking it, and those which nudge us to choose one soft drink, rather than another. We can find such remarkable neural correlates of psychological features and much more, yet we are unable to safely distinguish between a brain that hosts a universe and one that does not, between a fellow human who consciously exists and one who does not. The difference between being conscious and unconscious, after all, is the most important difference of all. Why it is so difficult to find it in the brain?

CHAPTER 4

MYSTERIES IN THE CRANIUM

As we have just seen, existential and philosophical issues aside, there are hard questions about consciousness that we are urgently called to address. The fact that we still feel uncertain when facing these questions may not be so surprising; perhaps, we haven't done all our homework. Why does the cortex support consciousness, but not the cerebellum, which has four times more neurons? Why does consciousness vanish during deep sleep, even though neurons remain active? How can the vivid experience of a dream be generated without interactions with the environment? Why does consciousness split if the corpus callosum is cut? These mysteries lie right in our own cranium; they involve concrete facts that are clearly discernible and have been for so decades. Maybe, such paradoxes, surprisingly ignored, in spite of the fact that they are so evident, represent challenges that should be faced in the first place.

The Cerebellum and the Thalamocortical System

Our cranium houses roughly 86 billion neurons, distributed across distinct structures, including the thalamocortical system and the cerebellum. The former, which is composed of the cerebral cortex and the thalamus, takes up most of the available space, while the latter is tucked away in the posterior cranial fossa, which is more or less at the level of the nape of the neck.

Indeed, this relatively small, extremely elegant, and compact structure contains the majority of our neurons: the cerebellum is home to roughly 70 billion neatly packed neurons, while the thalamocortical system has about only 16 billion [126]. As is to be expected, the cerebellum is rich in resources. Compared with the rest of the brain, its wiring is just as vast and intricate, it contains a cocktail of neurotransmitters that is just as rich, it is capable of exquisite plasticity and copes with an intense exchange of signals with the external world on both the input and output side [127]. It receives visual, acoustic, tactile, and various other signals, and emits motor commands that regulate many aspects of our behavior [128]. Even more, the cerebellum contains maps of the body and the outside space, and often shows selective activation during cognitive tasks and in relation to emotion. As if this were not enough, it is also strongly connected in both directions with the thalamus and indirectly with the cerebral cortex, especially the frontal cortex [129]. No doubt, the cerebellum is a marvel of biological intricacy just like the rest of the brain, with the difference that its phylogenetic history has even deeper, more ancient, roots.

The paradox is that the cerebellum, the largest neural structure in terms of the number of neurons, has very little to do with consciousness. There are certain tumors, which can invade it rapidly, threatening to spread to the rest of the brain; in these cases, the only option is to perform a very radical operation, and remove the cerebellum with its 70 billion neurons from the cranium and dump the whole lot in the surgical waste disposal unit. What are the consequences of such a drastic operation? An individual without a cerebellum is easily identifiable by the way he walks, gingerly and clumsily, with legs wide apart. He has difficulty in coordinating rapid movements, he shakes, and tends to articulate words syllable-by-syllable, sometimes with an explosive effect. Although such individuals may have obvious difficulty in coordinating their movements, their consciousness is surprisingly unaffected [130, 131]. In fact, the intensity of subjective experience in patients with cerebellar lesions does not seem to change and they continue to perceive the external world as before, with the same vividness and wealth of detail. Through forms, colors, sounds, smells, tastes, pain, emotions, and thoughts, the extraordinary variety of consciousness survives intact. A paradigmatic example is the remarkable story of a 24-year-old female patient from China [132]. The woman was admitted to the hospital after complaining of dizziness, nausea, and vomiting for about 1 month. Her mother reported to the caregivers that the woman's speech was unintelligible until the age of 6, and that she learned to walk only at the age of 7. For the rest of the time, she had led a seemingly normal life. At the time of admission, she was married with a daughter. The neurological examination revealed that she could cooperate and fully orient herself. Her word comprehension and expression were intact and she had no sign of aphasia, only a mild voice tremor, with slurred pronunciation and a harsh voice quality. The doctors gave her a MR scan and found that there was no cerebellum at all in her skull (complete cerebellar agenesis; Figure 4.1). She lacked 80% of her neurons, but she was definitely conscious.

The truth of the matter is that the cerebellum receives and processes visual and acoustic signals, and much more besides, it performs remarkable computations, but it is blind and deaf. The cerebellum is very good at playing piano, driving cars, and skiing, but has very little feeling to call its own. Thus, when it is surgically removed, consciousness remains. It is a 70 billion neurons zombie! We have not, however, yet discovered *why* it is a zombie. We know the cerebellum inside out, synapse after synapse, neuron after neuron; we can draw its basic circuitry on a blackboard, yet

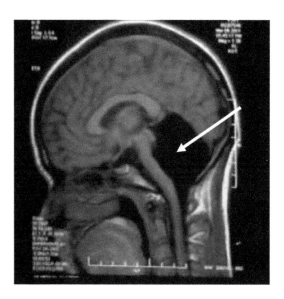

Figure 4.1 A conscious life, without a cerebellum. A T1-weighted sagittal MRI reveals that there is no recognizable cerebellar structure and the posterior fossa (indicated by the white arrow) is filled by cerebrospinal fluid. The patient was diagnosed with complete primary cerebellar agenesis, but had a normal life except for dizziness and nausea at the time of admission.

Reproduced from Carla Martins and Helena Hůlková, Neuroinflammation, mitochondrial defects and neurodegeneration in mucopolysaccharidosis III type C mouse model, *Brain*, 138 (2), pp. 336–355, https://doi.org/10.1093/brain/awu355 © 2015, Oxford University Press.

we cannot answer this basic question. This fact alone should be enough to justify the blackest pessimism.

If the cerebellum has so little relevance to consciousness, it stands to reason that the thalamocortical system, or at least parts of it, must instead be quite important and, indeed, all those unfortunate patients described in Chapter 3, "Brain Islands," are mute witnesses to this basic fact. A large lesion to the thalamocortical system can leave the patient an empty shell [30]. The relevance of this system is demonstrated not only by the irreversible eclipse of consciousness when its architecture is completely destroyed, but also by the consequences that result from focal lesions to specific regions of the cortex. For example, lesions in certain regions of the temporal lobes of the cerebral cortex will eliminate our acoustic experience, while damage to the occipital lobes may obliterate visual experiences. Smaller lesions may create lacunae in very specific aspects of our consciousness, while leaving the rest intact. If, for example, a tumor, heart attack, or surgical operation causes damage to visual area V5 in the visual cortex, the perception of motion will disappear, while other aspects of vision, such as the capacity to perceive form and color, will continue to function as before. Vice versa, if an area adjacent to visual area V5 is damaged, the perception of color, for example, will disappear, but the perception of motion will be unimpaired.

So why do the neurons of the thalamocortical system play a crucial role in determining subjective experience, while those of the cerebellum do not? It cannot be a question of sheer numbers, of how many neurons there are, or how many synapses; nor how many neurotransmitters or other molecules; nor is it a question of receiving impulses from the senses or the ability to influence motor activities. In all these aspects, the cerebellum can hold its own and more against the cerebral cortex. There is nothing here that would justify the dramatic difference in the effect on the capacity for experience following removal of the cerebellum (none) and of the thalamocortical system (consciousness is extinguished). Why does the cerebellum, with all its biological marvels, have no impact on consciousness, while the thalamocortical system does? Put the question to leading neuroanatomists and neurophysiologists; search for the answer on the stands of the Neuroscience Meeting, in the pages of the numerous texts on neurobiology and philosophy of mind. Nothing. Not even the shadow of an explanation. It is almost as if no one had ever asked the question; as if the question itself were so trivial as not to merit an answer. The reality, however, is very different. The simple fact that the thalamocortical system contains the physical substrate of consciousness and the cerebellum does not is of vital importance and should throw light on the biological basis of consciousness. These two structures represent a unique control experiment: they share many characteristics, but they are worlds apart when it comes to subjective experience. A very good vantage point from which to examine the fundamental differences between conscious and unconscious matter.

Asleep, Awake

An ancient theological tradition held that is not possible to list God's attributes as He is not subject to the limitations of our imagination. Therefore, it is preferable to specify what God is not, rather than what He is (in Latin, *via negationis*). This could be applied equally effectively to consciousness, as it is easier to specify what it is not, rather than what it is, at least until such time that a scientific explanation of the phenomenon is found. Today, a generally acceptable pre-scientific definition of consciousness could be that it is all that disappears when we fall into a dreamless sleep. In fact, when we sink into sleep early in the night the entire universe disappears, at least as far as we are concerned.

At first glance, it may look relatively simple to understand what is responsible for this nightly interruption of our conscious existence. Indeed, at the beginning of the last century the question did not seem to present any major difficulties; it was generally accepted that the brain shut down during the hours of sleep. The nerve cells needed a break to restore their energy after the stress of processing stimuli from the external world, programing movements, listening and speaking, and worrying about survival during the waking hours. Therefore, it was not surprising that consciousness, that trusty companion of wakefulness, should take a break, too.

Research studies put paid to this notion, showing that the brain is not silenced at all during sleep. At least, not in the way it was thought it did. We now know, too, that the majority of neurons in the cerebral cortex are just as active during sleep as they are during our waking hours. It may seem strange, but this is a relatively recent discovery. Until 15 years ago, with some rare exceptions, no-one had carefully compared the number of impulses spontaneously fired during sleep with those fired during wakefulness. For many reasons, historical, technical, or maybe just a question of scientific "vogues," the brain's spontaneous activity was considered to be less interesting than its reactions to sensory stimuli. Whatever the reasons, the fact is that, at the turn of the millennium, science knew a lot about how the neurons in the visual cortex produce electrical impulses when the retina is stimulated by horizontal lines, vertical lines, oblique lines, moving lines, intermittent flashing chessboard patterns, faces, landscapes, and much more besides, but much less about what these same neurons do when they are left to their own devices. A few scientists, however, notably among them Mircea Steriade, an old-school physiologist who observed the activity of cortical neurons far into his old age (80 years!) in a small laboratory at the University of Quebec, were curious to know. Thanks to their efforts we now know that if a cortical neuron fires on average 10–20 times/s when a person is awake, it will fire more or less the same number of times during deep sleep [89, 113] (Figure 4.2).

The neurons of the sleeping brain are constantly on the move. So, the question is why does consciousness fade during NREM sleep, even when neural activity does not? Why is it that when we wake someone from deep NREM sleep, especially early in the night, and ask them to report "anything that was going through your mind just before waking up" they will often say that they were not there, they were "coming out of nowhere, out of nothingness, as if I didn't exist" [115, 133].

As we said before, this fading of consciousness, consciousness that dwindles into oblivion is not accompanied by a commensurate decline in neural activity. There is a difference in how the neurons fire, certainly. The most significant difference seems to be that, during NREM sleep, the sequences of impulses emitted by the neurons become intermittent [88]. To a certain extent, scientists are now familiar with the mechanisms that are responsible for this phenomenon; what happens during NREM sleep is that the longer neurons remain depolarized and active, the more likely they are to precipitate into a hyperpolarized down-state—a complete cessation of synaptic activity that can last for a tenth of a second or more—after which they revert

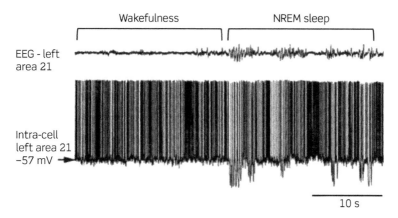

Figure 4.2 Cortical neurons are active during NREM sleep. The top trace represents depth-EEG activity recorded from area 21 in the cat's cerebral cortex during a spontaneous transition from wakefulness to sleep. The bottom trace is the intracellular activity recorded from a pyramidal neuron in the same area. During sleep the neuronal membrane may transiently become hyperpolarized (down-states), but average firing rates are comparable to wakefulness.

to another activated up-state [134, 135]. As we shall see later, this tendency of cortical neurons to fall into a silent hyperpolarized period after an initial activation is called bistability and appears to be due to depolarization-dependent potassium currents, which increase with the amount of prior activation. This phenomenon is evidently relevant, but why a person's universe should disappear due to the opening of potassium channels and a few hundred milliseconds of neuronal hyperpolarization remains a mystery.

Once again, there is no point in searching for the definitive answer to this enigma in the classic literature on neurobiology. It isn't there. Once again, we have come up against a situation of distinct opposites (a state of full consciousness, and being unconscious or almost so). Once again, we have an excellent control experiment to hand; the same physical architecture (nobody is destroying neurons or cutting connections in the cerebral cortex upon falling asleep) can switch from a conscious universe to dull matter and this depends on small changes in how the membranes of neurons are functioning. There has to be an explanation for this and it is definitely worth looking for.

Dreaming

Consciousness is not an exclusive privilege of wakefulness. The flame of consciousness can flare up in the witching hours and illuminate a universe that is completely disconnected from the external reality. This is probably the most interesting neurophysiological experiment of all. If we wake a person later in the night or in the early hours of the morning, what he will have to say about what is going on in his mind is probably not so very different to what he would say in his waking hours. These reports are especially frequent when subjects are awoken during a phase of sleep called rapid eye movement (REM; because it is characterized by rapid eye movements) [136]. Awakening from REM sleep yields reports of conscious experience 80–90% of the time and, especially in the early hours of the morning; the percentage is close to 100%, which is, of course, the report rate of wakefulness [137]. Dreams are long and complicated experiences, rich in vivid perceptions and emotions, which may take the form of a story:

> [...] I wake up and it is very early, maybe dawn has just broken because the light is milky and everything is silent . . . probably everyone in the house is still asleep. I get up and go into the kitchen; I see a light coming from the veranda. I go out onto the balcony and look outside. The usual landscape is transformed, everything is crystal . . . trees, houses, even the air. [. . .] Now the light is clearer and the facets of the crystal landscape reflect the light. I stand there, wide-eyed, looking at it. Everything is so beautiful. I feel both perturbed and happy at the same time. It was as if I had been sucked into the landscape, I felt I was a part of those crystals that I could see outside.

These sentences are taken from a dream narrated by a 9-year old girl. Sometimes the experiences we live in the dream world are just as vivid as those of wakefulness, sometimes even more so. Psychologists dedicate entire tomes to illustrating the differences between the mental activity that occurs during dreams and while awake, rather like cinema critics who write essays on the differences between the neo-realist and fantastic phases of Fellini's works. For our purposes, however, the similarities in these states are more important than the differences, because in both cases the director is the same—the conscious brain. When we dream we see forms, colors and movements, exactly as we do when we are awake. It is true, our critical sense is rather blunted and we tend to accept strange happenings as being completely normal, but we can count on our five senses (with the possible exception of the sense of smell) just as in our waking hours. The fundamental difference, which is truly astounding, is that when we dream our brain functions in complete autonomy. Especially during REM sleep, inputs from the environment are blocked somewhere in the sensory cortex, whereas the output from motor cortex are blocked on their way to the muscles, leading to a temporary paralysis [138]. The brain sees without the retina, walks without legs, disconnected from nerves and muscles. So, we are left with the fact that dreaming, traditionally belittled by science as being unpredictable and ephemeral, on the contrary, has a crucial scientific value. Consciousness is not produced through interaction with the external world *here and now*, it exists in the brain! If that brain were to be disconnected from its nerves, extracted from the cranium and kept alive in a bath of oxygen and sugar, the dream would continue, rich and bizarre as before, unpredictable as always. Just as if nothing untoward had happened.

Other Facts to be Explained

The paradoxes regarding the relationship between the thalamocortical system and the cerebellum, wakefulness, deep sleep, and dreaming throw an unrelenting light on basic facts that we cannot explain still and indicate where we should be directing our efforts in the first place. However, there are more enigmas to be investigated and solved.

Take the retina, for example. Just as the other sense organs, it determines what we perceive visually at any given moment, but its neural activity does not appear to contribute directly to conscious experience. While the cells of the retina can distinguish between light and dark, and transmit this information to the visual cortex, their continuously changing discharge profile does not correspond at all to the stable visual field that we perceive [139]. In other words, what the retina sees is not what we see. In addition to that, it is well known that retinal blindness in adults does not prevent recall of colors, or imagining or dreaming in vivid color. How can this be explained?

The discharge activity of the long neural chains that connect the cerebral cortex to the muscles is necessary to obtain the behavioral responses normally associated with conscious experience, but does not make any contribution to consciousness. We have already seen that patients with LIS caused by lesions to the ventral portion of the pons, completely paralyzed with the exception of the muscles of the eyes, which can sometimes perform vertical movements, are nonetheless fully conscious. We have also seen that, when we dream, we are conscious, but paralyzed. Last, but not least, we have seen that even vast lesions to the central motor system do not affect consciousness. Again, the question is ... why?

The neural activations which take place in the basal ganglia, a voluminous subcortical structure tightly connected to the thalamocortical system, are important for the production of language, through motor sequences [140]. Their activity provide a crucial drive for motor outputs [141], but the neural processes that occur inside these structures do not appear to be necessary for consciousness [142, 143]. So the question once more is ... why?

The activating systems of the brain stem, which we have seen to be fundamental for staying awake, act in many ways as an on/off switch that can influence the global state of the thalamocortical system [144] and, consequently, of the state of consciousness. This explains why lesions of dysfunctions to these structures can cause a person to fall into a coma. On the other hand, we have seen that the VS/UWS patients with an intact brain stem, but a severely damaged thalamocortical system open their eyes and look awake, but remain unconscious. Why are the neurons of the brainstem activating system critical for maintaining a state of wakefulness, but at the same time do not appear to contribute directly to conscious experience?

If the thalamocortical system is split, consciousness splits. Some epileptic patients used to be subjected to a callosotomy, in which the corpus callosum, a wide, flat bundle of 200 million fibers that connects the two hemispheres of the brain, is severed. The rationale for this quite radical intervention was to preserve at least one hemisphere from the spread of the frequent seizures originating in the confraternal one. After surgery, patients reported a better quality of life, in spite of a really radical change.

As shown by extensive research, the two split hemispheres each house a different conscious individual [145]. How is this possible?

Psychophysiological studies show that 200–500 ms elapse before a sensory stimulus is perceived consciously [146]. Why is this? Why does it appear that neural activity only contributes to consciousness at certain temporal intervals and not at others?

These facts are in front of our eyes; they are tangible both clinically and experimentally, and offer plenty of paradoxes to think about. Will we simply need to collect more data to come up with an answer to these paradoxes, develop new technical marvels to dig deeper in the brain? Should we look for a yet unidentified gene, an unknown molecule, a special neuron, or a rare diamond still hiding inside the cranium? Maybe not. Perhaps, what is really missing at this stage is a theory—a fundamental, principled approach to consciousness—what it is and what it may take to have it. After all, there are precedents in the history of biology. Take evolution by natural selection—there were many, well-known observations in support of the theory before Darwin published his *Origins of the Species by Means of Natural Section*. The individual variations within each species were clearly visible, as was the continuity between the species. Breeders had been selecting hereditary characteristics through cross-breeding with almost scientific precision for centuries. A large amount of suggestive information was there. What was missing was a theoretical principle, a key to combine the available data.

One of the fundamental principles of reason, maybe its very root, is the Principle of Sufficient Reason. In Latin this is stated as *nihil est sine ratione cur potius sit quam non sit*. Nothing happens without a reason. There has to be an explanation as to why something is the way it is and not otherwise. Why some physical mechanisms, but not others, should be associated with consciousness? There has to be a reason behind the paradoxes identified in this chapter, unless consciousness has nothing to do with the brain, or we decide to waive all reason.

CHAPTER 5

A THEORETICAL PRINCIPLE

Starting with Galileo Galilei, scientists have done their utmost to eliminate all traces of subjectivity from the study of Nature. All scientific theories start from the observation of the objective properties of natural phenomena, those which presumably do not depend on the perspective of the observer. The study of these objective properties provides the founding principles in physics, chemistry, biology, and so on. Consciousness, however, is different. What makes it different is its relation with the scientific observer. The physical process we are studying here, unlike all the other processes and objects that can be described in objective terms, involves ourselves as subjective conscious observers; hence, we cannot exclude ourselves from the analysis. This requires a radical change in perspective. In his *Discourse on the Method of Rightly Conducting the Reason, and Seeking Truth in the Sciences* [6] Descartes took his famous *cogito ergo sum* as a basis. This consisted in acknowledging the primacy of consciousness. He famously argued that, while it is always possible that we might be mistaken about the nature of objects in the external world, of one thing we can be certain—that our subjective experience exists. This is the ground truth and to formulate a theoretical principle about consciousness one can only start from this "zeroth" axiom—that subjective experience exists.

The theory that will guide us through the rest of this book addresses the problem of consciousness in a new way. The integrated information theory (IIT) does not start from the brain and ask how it could give rise to experience. Indeed, as long as one starts from the brain —in effect trying to squeeze consciousness out of matter, the problem of consciousness may be not only hard, but almost impossible to solve [7]. We have seen several examples of this difficulty in the first part of this book. Instead, IIT starts from the essential phenomenal properties of experience, and infers postulates about the characteristics that are required of its physical substrate [147, 148]. In essence, the theory is grounded on the best available data on consciousness: the fundamental structure of experience, as we—healthy, adult individuals—know it. Based on this, it makes an inference to the best explanation: a general hypothesis about what kind mechanisms, in the physical world, may account for this phenomenological structure and what may not. Then, it proposes a measure to test hypothesis, make predictions and novel inferences.

In this chapter, we will introduce IIT in a rather light-weighted manner, thus we will try to avoid equations, and focus on the minimal set of principles[1] that are necessary to address the practical problems we have encountered so far. Why is the thalamocortical system crucial for consciousness, but not the cerebellum with all its neurons? Why does consciousness fade, while neurons remain active during sleep? What should we try to measure at the bedside of patients? Where do we start when we are called to find out whether someone feels pain, even though it may be unresponsive, or instead whether something is merely a zombie that acts as if it felt pain without actually feeling anything? Finally, what makes this small object that I can hold on the palm of my hand so different and special?

From Phenomenology to the Physical Substrate of Consciousness

A simple way to introduce IIT is to summarize it as follows:

> A physical system has subjective experience to the extent that it is capable of integrating information.

This statement about the physical substrates of consciousness, which may seem at a first reading to be cryptic and abstract, is actually rather immediate. It derives from two fundamental phenomenological properties of experience:

- conscious experience is informative;
- conscious experience is integrated.

---

1 The full set of axioms and postulates of IIT can be found in [149].

These two properties are so essential and embedded in the second-by-second flow of our daily existence that we typically take them for granted. To see them it may be useful to engage in a couple of thought experiments.

Information

Imagine facing a large blank screen that extends beyond your visual field. So does a small photodiode—a small electrical circuit with a variable resistance that changes with exposure to light. The photodiode gives an "on" signal when the current exceeds a certain value, and an "off" signal when it is below that value. All you have to do is to say "light" when the screen is white and "dark" when it turns black, which it does every few seconds or so. Clearly, both you and the photodiode can perform this simple task equally well. Clearly, you were alternately aware of light and dark. The question is: was the photodiode as aware of light and dark as you were? The photodiode performed perfectly, perhaps better than you did (it does not get distracted), but was it aware of light and dark? The question does not even sound relevant. You can buy the photodiode for a few dollars at the electronics department and you can crush it under your foot with no qualms. Why should you have the benefit of experience, whereas the photodiode, who behaved just like you during the test, should be devoid of it?

Forget the idea that it is being made of biological matter that makes the difference. Remember that the cells of the retina and the cerebral cortex, which fire when you see light, are also photodiodes, only composed of carbon, oxygen, hydrogen, and nitrogen. Forget the idea that it is just a difference in the size and the intricacy of the circuits they form because you know that there are structures inside your brain, such as the cerebellum, which are composed of myriads of elements arranged in complicated ways, but are still irrelevant for subjective experience. Then, why me, but not the photodiode? Recall the principle of sufficient reason: *nihil est sine ratione cur potius sit quam non sit*. There must be a reason.

Let us continue with the thought experiment. As you are absorbed in these thought, the screen is flooded with light again, but this time it is a uniform red light. You are faced with a dilemma. You were told to distinguish between light and dark, no-one said anything about color. Should you shout "Red!" or say there has been a mistake? At the same time, the change in the intensity of light has already altered the resistance of the photodiode, which now signals "On." After a few seconds, the screen turns blue, then green, yellow, and brown. Each time you have a different experience. Then the screen suddenly shows a beautiful painting, then another one, first post-modern, then impressionist, then a splendid example of early renaissance art, then an incomprehensible representation of cows in the cubist style. The number of possible paintings is countless. Then you see a human figure, then another, changing dress, face, and expression; and then the screen begins displaying some movie frames, and then, you begin to think, every possible frame from every possible movie . . . Clearly, for each one of these images, you would have a specific experience, different from any other, but what about the photodiode? Flooded with countless images on the screen, the photodiode would have just entered one of two states: "on" or "off," depending on the amount of light. Nothing more, nothing less. So, this is the fundamental difference! During the first experiment, each time you called out "dark!" you were not only singling out dark from "light!," but from millions of billions of other possible states of affairs; when the photodiode called "off," it was just singling out "off," from "on," the only other state available to it (Figure 5.1).

Claude Shannon, the "father of the information theory," defined information as a reduction of uncertainty [150]. This reduction depends on the repertoire of possible states that are ruled out once a system enters one particular state. For example, if a coin falls with the heads side upward, just one alternative is excluded, but when a dice falls with the three dot face upwards more uncertainty is eliminated, that is more information is generated; for example, we know that the dice did not fall with the one, two, four, five and six dot faces uppermost. Information is measured in *bits* and is equal to the logarithm of the possible alternatives. In the case of the coin, which has only two alternatives, the information can be expressed as 1 bit [$\log_2(2) = 1$], while in the case of the dice with its six potential states, the formula is 2.58 bit [$(\log_2(6) = 2.58$].

Returning to the experiment once again, even when we have the simplest of experiences, such as when we see pure dark, the repertoire of possibilities is immense, as is the amount of information (expressed in bit) that is specified by the brain in fraction of a second (Figure 5.1).

The darkness that we perceive is dark because it differs in a particular way from other innumerable conscious states: pure light, a starry sky pure red, pure blue, nuances of color without end, half red, half blue, an infinite combination of objects, paintings, landscapes, human beings,

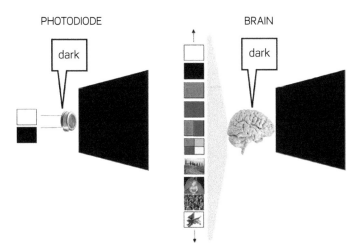

Figure 5.1 Information. When the photodiode signals "off" it only specifies "dark," rather than "light", corresponding to one "bit" of information. On the other hand, when we report "dark" our brain specifies a particular state of affair, one out of a countless number of alternatives, corresponding to a large amount of information.

Photodiode: © OSRAM GmbH. and Jesada Sabai/Shutterstock.com

Brain: © Jesada Sabai/Shutterstock.com

words, phrases, tastes, smells, emotions, thoughts, dreams, fantasies, memories, hopes, desires, and any combination of these, and yet more again. Information, the ability to differentiate between an almost inexhaustible set of alternatives, is a fundamental aspect of our conscious experience. There must be an intrinsic mechanism for this. Thus, we can write down the first principle and ensuing postulate:

Consciousness experience is rich in information

Thus,

the physical substrate of consciousness must be highly differentiated— that is, it must be able to generate a vast repertoire of states

In other words, the physical substrate of consciousness has to be much more than a photodiode, a coin, or a dice. A diamond cut to show billions of billions of facets would be a better comparison.

Integration

However, information alone is worthless if it is not integrated. To see this, let us go back in the room and replace our opponent with a digital camera with a resolution of one megapixel, instead of the photodiode. The sensor of the camera is composed of a million photodiodes arranged on a regular grating behind the lens, which as in the previous experiment respond to variations in the intensity of light with a corresponding variation in the resistance of the current. Each element of the sensor signals "on" or "off" according to the presence or absence of light in the corresponding area by the other side of the lens. Now the situation is very different: the sensor of the camera is able to provide differentiated responses to an immense number of scenes. When you aim the camera to a new scene, to a blank wall, a red wall, a white wall, a blue wall, a wall painted half in red and half in blue, a face, a different face, a landscape, a different landscape and so on, the combination of "on" and "off" photodiodes will change. Assuming, for the sake of simplicity, that we are dealing with a black and white camera, the sensor can provide different responses to $2^{1,000,000}$ different states, which is perhaps comparable to the repertoire of potential conscious states.

So, does this mean that the digital camera is a conscious entity? Surely not! Then, how can the ability to distinguish among billions of states that set us apart from the photodiode in the first experiment, be crucial for consciousness if it does not distinguish us from a commercial camera? Again, let's appeal to the principle of sufficient reason and take a closer look at the camera: we can hold it in our hands and it appears to be a single entity, but in reality its unity is just an illusion—an error of perspective. The unity of the camera is only in the eye of the beholder, but there is no actual reason to consider a collection of photodiodes as single entity. In fact, this is an ontological error. We are attributing existence to something that does not exist for itself. If we consider the camera by its intrinsic perspective, it immediately disintegrates in millions of parts. Each photodiode of the sensor array is perfectly independent from the others. There are no causal interactions between the elements of the sensors, by design. If we were to cut the sensor of the camera with a thin blade in two, with 500,000 photodiodes in the right half and 500,000 in the left half, what would change? The answer is "nothing!" The camera would continue to function as before, capturing images and transmitting them correctly. Even if you cut the video-camera into four, 16, or a million parts, the result would still be the same, because the photodiodes function independently one from the other. Every one of the million photodiodes will go on reporting its own separate dot (Figure 5.2, left panel). There has never been, nor will there ever be, any interaction between them, because they are separate entities. The truth of the matter is that the casing of the camera does not contain one single entity capable of accessing billions and billions of states, but just a collection of 1 million single entities, each capable of accessing one of two states, corresponding to 1 bit of information. Indeed, the camera does not have any more information than the sum of its parts. Therefore, at least with respect to information, there is no need to invoke the camera above its parts. We might as well drop it from the list of existing entities and stick with a million photodiodes.

What if, instead, we take the same thin blade and cut the brain in two? Would nothing change, as with the camera? For example, would the visual field continue to be perceived as a single image? Not at all. As was mentioned earlier, until recently neurosurgeons used to cut the corpus callosum to treat severe cases of drug-resistant epilepsy, separating the hemispheres to prevent an interhemispheric spread of the epileptic activity. This neurosurgical procedure produced a special condition, the so-called split-brain. Split-brain patients were able to return to a normal life fairly soon after the operation without too many problems, and the frequency and spread of seizures were much reduced. The side effect of this treatment was that the patient was no longer one patient, but two. One would see the right side of the world, and the other the left side, but neither would see the whole image.

It is now clear that complete callosotomy results in the paradox of two separate conscious experiences sharing the same skull. The resident of the left hemisphere may have much better language and reasoning skills, whereas the one of the right hemisphere may be stronger at drawing, but hardly speaks at all. Crucially, the talkative left hemisphere is largely unaware of what its right twin sees, touches, or draws. Similarly, the right hemisphere has no explicit idea of what the left one hears, reads, or says. Although some cross-talk is still possible through thin bundles of subcortical fibers passing from one hemisphere to the other, the right hand literally does not know what the left hand is doing. This interesting condition was thoroughly investigated by Roger Sperry

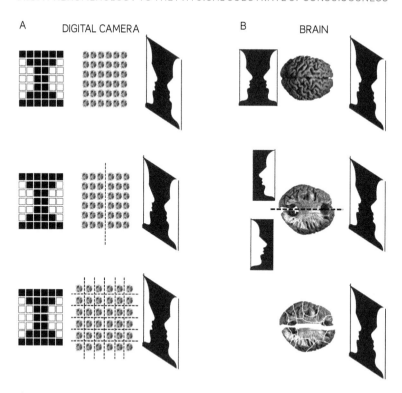

Figure 5.2 Integration. Although to an external observer the sensor array of a digital camera appears to be a single entity, it is a collection of independent entities, the individual photodiodes, when it is examined by an intrinsic perspective. In fact, the sensor can be cut into two, four, or all its parts without impacting on its function. Indeed, by an intrinsic perspective what exists are only the individual photodiodes and their output is unchanged. The brain functions differently; when it enters one of the countless states available it does so as a single, integrated system. This also means that we can only be in one conscious state at a time. In the vase-face picture, we either see two faces or the vase (a). When the brain is divided into two, consciousness is divided into two also, as shown by split-brain patients. The conscious subject in the right hemisphere will see the face on the left, and vice versa. When the brain is cut into many parts, such as when connections are severed by diffuse axonal injury, consciousness is lost (b).

Figure 5.2a: EUSKALANATO/Flickr (CC BY-SA 2.0)

and Michael Gazzaniga in laboratory conditions [145, 151]. They found that both hemispheres have their own private experiences, their own very private thoughts, personality, and motivation to act, all of which is inaccessible for the other hemisphere. Usually, split-brain patients continued their existence without any major difficulties and people around them would hardly notice a change. Indeed, the two hemispheres had grown up together, playing and working together, sharing the same world, millisecond-by-millisecond, for decades. Thus, they get along pretty well, much better than any couple of identical twins and they seem like one single individual to the external observer. However, from the intrinsic point of view there is nothing it is like to be "one" split-brain patient.

Now what would happen if we were to cut the brain into four, eight, 16, or a million parts, to the point of severing each of the fibers that connect the 100 billion neurons housed inside the casing of the skull? In theory, the cranium would be left with a huge collection of biological photodiodes, each having one bit (or slightly more) of information. A mass of binary elements for which dark would mean nothing more than one of two states.

What happens to consciousness in practice? A person involved in a car accident may experience deceleration from 100 km/h to 0 in the fraction of a second. The effect of such a change in speed to the brain can be totally devastating—ripping apart and disrupting the axons, those delicate fibers that connect the neurons to each other. Diffuse axonal injury, as this form of trauma is called, causes tissues of differing densities to slide over each other and stretch the axons that cross the junctions between the white and grey matter. Probably not all neurons will be separated from each other, but the result is shattering and in most cases result in loss of consciousness, that is, the result is a persistent VS/UWS [30].

We have seen that cutting the sensor of a camera into a million parts makes no difference as the camera was never a single entity in the first place, but cutting the brain into parts a makes huge difference. This points to a crucial distinction that is often neglected—the camera does not exist as such, while the brain is a single entity with billions and billions of states at its disposal. Since the brain generates each one of the particular shapes of experience as a single, integrated piece, it can only enter one state at a time. Here comes the second fundamental principle— each conscious experience is integrated, that is, indivisible, irreducible to its parts. As illustrated in Figure 5.2 (right panel), at any given moment we will perceive either the faces or the vase, it is impossible to see both at once. Nor will we ever see our left visual field separated from the right visual field unless our brain is divided into two, as in split-brain patients. Every second of our conscious life, every time we see a face or a vase, or a blue wall or red wall, and every time we close our eyes to the dark, our brain rifles through billions of possibilities and does so as a single entity. In the intact brain, information is for the system as a whole, above and beyond its parts.

Thus, we can write down the second principle and ensuing postulate:

Conscious experience is integrated

thus

the physical substrate of consciousness must constitute a single, integrated entity.

Combining the information postulate with the integration postulate, we derive the keystone of the theory:

a physical system has subjective experience to the extent that it is capable of integrating information

In essence, the central assumption of IIT is that these two fundamental properties of conscious experience—information and integration—rest on the coexistence of differentiation and integration, that is, on a unique balance between diversity and unity in the physical brain. This is a non-trivial assumption as, at first sight, it would seem that these two properties are extremely difficult to reconcile. They act as two forces working against each other. The more specialized the elements of a system are, the more difficult it is to make them interact and, consequently, integration will be extremely arduous. On the other hand, the stronger and more efficient the interaction between the elements, the more homogeneous their behavior will be and the overall level of differentiation within the system will be reduced. Loosely speaking, the coexistence of differentiation and integration is no easy matter in any walk of life, from the personal to the political, from the biological to the organization of human society, let alone in physical systems. Somehow, these two opposing forces have reached an improbable, optimal equilibrium somewhere in the matter of the brain. Now, this keystone may be falsified or validated by empirical evidence. To do this, the coexistence of information and integration has to be expressed in quantitative terms: a measure has to be found to quantify a system's capacity to integrate information.

Φ: Measuring Integrated Information

Methods have been developed for measuring the quantity of information that can be transmitted from a source to a receiver through a channel (such as the optical fibers used for Internet) and for measuring the quantity of information that can be stored on a physical support (such as the hard disk on a computer, for example), but there is still no way to measure a system's capacity for integrating information. What is needed is a method to quantify the amount of information that a system can generate as a whole, above and beyond its parts.

This is certainly no easy task, not least because science has developed measures for almost all physical phenomena, but still lacks a serious way to establish one key property of the objects of the universe, that is, whether they constitute an entity or not. When is an entity one entity? How can multiple elements be a single thing? A very simple question that has not yet been answered or, perhaps, it had not yet been asked, at least in scientific terms. To do so, IIT introduces a novel quantity, called Phi and denoted by the Greek letter Φ, which can be in principle applied to any physical system. The vertical bar of the Greek letter stands for information, while the circle indicates integration. The value of Φ is expressed in bits, the unit measure of information but, as we shall remark later, the term information is used very differently in IIT and in Shannon's classic theory of communication. While the idea behind Φ is simple enough, the actual calculation can be rather complex. As for the principles of IIT, we will outline the fundamental procedure underlying the quantification of integrated information in a simplified manner.[2]

The first fundamental tenet is that observation, in itself, is not sufficient to measure integrated information. As shown by the thought

2 A detailed description of the principles and of the mathematical framework for measuring Φ can be found in [148] and [149].

experiment about distinguishing light and dark, an external observer, say an alien researcher, would not have been able to detect the difference between a conscious human and a photodiode. By considering behavioral responses, he would have no means of knowing that, for the human brain, the experience of darkness excluded billions upon billions of other possible states, that darkness is not simply the absence of light, but also the absence of red, blue, a starry sky, a sound, of everything that humans can imagine and dream, and all the possible combinations of these innumerable states. These states could potentially have happened within the brain, but did not. This intrinsic repertoire is, in fact, what counts, what has to be measured. What we need to quantify here is very different from information as classically defined. For Shannon and for most neuroscientists, information is extrinsic and observational; it is assessed from the extrinsic perspective of an observer and it quantifies how accurately input signals can be decoded from the output signals transmitted across a noisy channel. Here, information is intrinsic and causal; it is assessed from the intrinsic perspective of a system based on the cause–effect repertoire generated by its internal mechanisms. In the light–dark experiment, in order to know that the brain was different from the photodiode, the alien researcher should have opened the black-box and perturbed the elements of each system in all possible ways. Then, he would have learned that, unlike the photodiode, the brain had an extremely differentiated set of internal mechanisms by which many different causes (perturbations) would have produced many different effects. So, the first general principle is that, above and beyond what the system is actually doing, one needs to explore its intrinsic potential, the size of the cause–effect repertoire that can be generated by its internal mechanisms. If many different perturbations reliably produce many specific effects—if differences make the difference within the system itself—we will know that any state generated within the system is highly informative to itself, even when all that the subject is doing is just signaling light or dark. Indeed, checking every possible counter factual by applying perturbations to the photodiode would have promptly revealed a trivially small intrinsic cause–effect repertoire, whereby all causes would have inevitably converged into a stereotypical response.

Now comes another challenge. Are we actually dealing with one entity or with a collection of separate mechanisms? How is it possible to establish whether a large number of specific responses to a large number of different perturbations are produced by one integrated system or by an aggregate of independent elements? What counts, according to IIT, is only the information that is irreducible to that specified by independent sub-systems. The basic idea is very simple—if partitioning a system makes no difference to the information it generates, there is no system to begin with. In practice, the amount of irreducible information is the one identified by the cruelest cut among all possible cuts. This is the cut that passes through the system's weakest link, the one that divides the system into its strongest parts—those that generate as much information as possible by themselves, leaving as little as possible for the whole.

Take the camera. Cutting the sensor chip in two, or in any other way, would make no difference to the information generated by its million photodiodes. Indeed, every cut would reveal a weakest link between the photodiodes, corresponding to 0 bit. It is thus immediately evident that the camera is not an entity from its own intrinsic perspective and the only irreducible information that one can measure is that generated by the individual photodiodes (Φ = 1 bit). Now consider the brain. In this case, all cuts would lead to a loss of information because neurons tend to be linked by effective connections. The brain as whole, then, can integrate information. However, parts of the brain may integrate more information than the whole brain itself. Indeed, one must consider any set of elements within a system—in this case, say, neurons—and measure how much information they integrate by finding their "minimum cut"— their weakest link—the one that determines to what extent they can be a single entity. In the end, within the brain, one will sooner or later find a particular set of neurons, a core for which the value of Φ is *maximal*. That complex of neurons—the one that is maximally integrated—will correspond to the neural substrate of consciousness, or so says IIT.

As a simple illustration, we will now apply these principles to a number of simple models composed of eight elements. Of course, these models cannot compare with the staggering numbers of the brain, but they do provide a concrete and hopefully accessible illustration of how the measure of Φ works.

Figure 5.3 shows, on the far left of the top row, a system composed of eight elements, representing neurons. Here, the elements interact in pairs, forming four modules that cannot interact, however. This gives the system a certain degree of differentiation as each element has very specific connections. Indeed, if the system is fully challenged, for example,

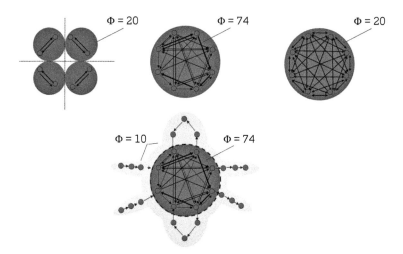

Figure 5.3 Four simplified models end the corresponding values of integrated information. The blue dots represent the elements (neurons) and the arrows the connections between them. For each model, the grey dark area represents the partition of the system with maximum Φ. In the lower panel, the light-grey area indicates the larger system with lower Φ and the dotted lines highlight the weak links.

by perturbing all its components in various combinations, a different response will be obtained each time. If element 1 is stimulated, element 2 will fire, if element 3 fires it will trigger element 4, and so on, resulting in a fairly elevated repertoire of states. However, it becomes soon obvious that this system is not integrated as there are cuts that reveal the absence of any interaction between the various modules (the presence of partitions yielding 0 bit); the system can be decomposed (actually, it does not exist) and its Φ value is low, because it can be reduced to the one of its individual modules.

On the far right of the top row there is another system, which clearly lays at the other end of the spectrum. This is a homogeneous system in which each element interacts with all the others, with no "weak links:" the system is integrated because all its elements interact with all the others. However, for this very reason the amount of information generated by the system will be low, since all elements will behave in the same way. This becomes obvious when the cause–effect repertoire is measured through an exhaustive set of perturbations. When element 1 is stimulated, all the other elements will be activated and the same global, stereotypical responses will be obtained for elements 2, 3, 4, 5, 6, 7, and 8, revealing that the system is, in fact, a single entity, but with a low repertoire of potential states. This minimal repertoire of states leads to a low Φ, even though the system is integrated. This shows that integration alone is not sufficient to obtain high Φ values, if the elements that compose the system are not able to engage in specific causal interactions.

The eight-element system in the middle of the top line balances the differentiation of the model to the left with the integration of the model to the right. In this case, different perturbations produce many specific effects within the system (high information). Yet there is no cut that can split the system into two parts without drastically decreasing the information generated by the system (high integration). Indeed, this system was created by a calculator that arranged the connections between the eight elements in all possible ways, until it found the highest value of Φ. Such an optimization process required several hours of computations, a time that rises exponentially if one searches for the best balance in larger systems. These three simple models show, in a rather intuitive way, how Φ can quantify the capacity for integrated information, which depends on the joint presence of differentiation and integration in the functional architecture of a system. They also provide a practical example of how the information captured by Φ is intrinsic, causal, and irreducible.

Now, in order to highlight another important property of this measure, let's examine one last system. The model depicted in the lower panel of Figure 5.3 is a mini-brain composed of 26 elements, which has been constructed by taking the system above ($\Phi = 74$) and adding six chains of three elements each. This is, indeed, a larger system whose elements are all engaged in some sort of interactions. In this case, no cut will result in zero bit of integrated information, because there will always be some effect, albeit minimal, among any of the partitions. Now, the question is whether a system of interacting elements that is simply larger will automatically integrate more information. What will Φ reveal in this case? Perturbation after perturbation and cut after cut, the analysis would mercilessly reveal a weak link. Indeed, there is a partition of the entire system, the one indicated by the dotted line, across which Φ is not zero (it is 10 bits), but is much lower than the information integrated by the smaller subset of system elements that form the system's core (74 bits). Therefore, from the point of view of integrated information, the extra elements in the chains add nothing whatsoever; there is no reason to take the larger system into consideration if it integrates less information than one of its subsets. After all, this is just a generalization of the extreme case represented by the camera. There is no point in considering the sensor of the camera as it integrates less information than the individual photodiodes. What really counts is the subset of elements that integrate more information than its subsystems (including its elements taken singly) and more than the any larger system of which it is a part.

In metaphorical terms, one could say that the measure Φ is like Occam's razor—whatever is not necessary and does not add anything is automatically eliminated. It cuts into the heart of the system, peeling and dropping, until it reaches the core where integrated information is maximal. The maximum density of diversity in a unity or, in more technical terms, a maximum of irreducible intrinsic cause–effect power. This improbable balance is what a physical system should have to account for the richness and unity of subjective experience. That which, at least in theory, can make light luminous and darkness dark.

CHAPTER 6

REAPPRAISING THE STUFF IN OUR HEAD

So far, we have only posed questions. Now, it is time to start the return leg of the journey in search of explanations and answers guided by a theoretical principle. We leave behind the photodiodes, the camera, and the simple eight-element systems, and return to biological matter. The first stop is within the cranium, where we will try to unravel the tangle of neurons that is tucked in there. If the theoretical foundations are anywhere near the mark, consciousness will shine brighter where there are complexes with higher Φ.

Just to Keep Our Hand In

Before starting on the brain, let's have a quick look at the other organs, the ones located outside the skull, so as to leave nothing to chance. For example, one would like to test whether some sophisticated biological systems, such as the liver and the heart, may or may not contain complexes capable of high Φ.

The liver is organized in such a way as to efficiently conduct various biochemical reactions to construct and eliminate molecules, but its cells do not have strong means of communicating effectively, one with the other, on a large scale. Looking at it through the lens of the integrated information theory, the liver is not a single object, but is divided into four lobes, which are, in turn, composed of a myriad of microscopic lobules that are functionally independent, one from the other. Thus, the liver looks very much like the modular system with minimal Φ that we investigated in the preceding chapter (Figure 5.3, upper left).

If we were to cut the liver into two or more parts (with microsurgical precision, obviously!) it would continue to function effectively, like the split sensor of the video-camera.

The heart, on the other hand, is a single thing. The cells of the myocardium not only produce electrical impulses like neurons, they also communicate reciprocally through connections (electrical synapses) that are stronger, faster, and more direct than those that connect brain cells. These connections permit a synchronous contraction, so that at each heart beat a powerful wave of electrical impulses floods through the entire organ, activating hundreds of millions of cells in an orderly manner and in a fraction of a second. Looking at the heart from this point of view it certainly seems to be an integrated system and if we were to cut it into two parts, there is no doubt that its functionality would change drastically. However, although the heart is definitely a unitary object, by and large it lacks differentiation. With the exception of a handful of conduction fibers with specific arrangement, the cells of the heart are interconnected in a highly homogeneous and stereotypical way. Every cell of the myocardium is directly connected to its neighbor; the wave of electrical activity floods through the heart like the ripples a stone causes when thrown into water. It makes no difference where the first stimulus takes place, the final result is always the same; all the cells in the heart will activate and contract. This is good because we can use simple pace-makers and defibrillators to save lives. On the other hand, as we saw in Chapter 5, "A Theoretical Principle," a system that reacts to different perturbations by generating stereotypical, all-or-nothing responses cannot integrate information and its Φ is minimal (Figure 5.3, upper right). Indeed, in spite of its unity, clinical, and symbolic relevance, the heart—just like the liver—can be replaced by a machine or transplanted without any fear of moving consciousness from one body to another.

The Cerebellum and the Thalamocortical System

Ok, this was just a digression, an exercise to become familiar with the tools we have at hand. The liver and the heart were relatively easy to analyze, but now comes the brain and the going gets tougher. We are faced with 100 billion nerve cells, connected by an estimated one quadrillion synapses (numbers that can dwarf the Milky Way). The cramped estate in the cranium offers multiple opportunities for communication and it houses structures with an architectural intricacy that, as far as we know, is unrivalled in the universe, all in the space of two fists. This is where we encounter the first major paradox, however; the vast majority of the neurons and synapses that make up the encephalon have little to do with consciousness.

You will remember that the cerebellum, which has many more neurons (70 billion) and synapses than the thalamocortical system, can be removed in its entirety from the cranium without impacting the content and vividness of consciousness [131, 152]. Thus, subjectively, the contribution of the cerebellum to the capacity for consciousness is irrelevant. Instead, many kinds of lesions of the remaining 16 billion neurons, the ones in the thalamocortical system can lead to the irreversible annihilation of consciousness [30]. This is one of the most relevant pieces of evidence in our possession and is of fundamental importance for the integrated information theory.

Let's take a moment to recap. IIT states that conscious experience as we know it is associated with the presence of complexes with high Φ. Thus, if it was to be discovered that, in terms of their capacity for integrated information, there is no significant difference between the thalamocortical system and cerebellum, then the theory would have to be discarded and there would be no point in continuing our quest. Therefore, before proceeding it is necessary to examine the differences between the thalamocortical system and the cerebellum through the lens of the theory.

The cerebellum receives a plethora of impulses that transmit visual and acoustic signals from the eyes and ears, vestibular signals from the organs of balance, somatosensory signals from the receptors in the skin, muscles, and tendons, and a variety of signals from other parts of the brain regarding movements that are being executed or will be executed in the near future. Each signal is transmitted to a module of the cerebellar cortex, which takes the form of a cloak of neurons that covers the surface of the cerebellum, not unlike how the cerebral cortex covers the surface of the cerebrum. Inside the neural circuits of each module, the incoming electrical impulses are added, subtracted, multiplied, compared, and processed, until finally a signal is emitted from the cerebellum.

At a first glance, this is not very different from what happens in the thalamocortical system. The same types of signal regarding sight, hearing, touch, and movement are sent to specialized centers in the cerebral cortex. Here, as in the cerebellum, they are added, subtracted, multiplied, compared, and processed. Each module of the cerebral cortex then emits a response through output nerve fibers.

Simply on the basis of the vast variety of signals that both the cerebellum and the thalamocortical system receive and process, it can safely be said that both structures are highly differentiated. In fact, if we return for a moment to the room of the photodiode experiment, we can see that the neurons of the cerebellar cortex and those of the cerebral cortex produce specific responses to different stimuli, acoustic, visual, tactile, movement, acceleration, and so on [127]. However, in spite of their similarity in this exquisite degree of functional differentiation, there is a radical difference between the cerebellum and the thalamocortical system—a difference that could easily be missed if we did not have a principle at hand.

Now, we remember the sharp blade that cut the sensor of the camera into pieces and what it revealed. Back in the morgue, with the cerebellum in one hand and the cerebrum in the other, we pull the two hemispheres of the cerebral cortex and those of the cerebellum apart to see if they are connected by a bundle of fibers. It feels rather like butchery, but in this case, the means are justified by the result—the two hemispheres of the cerebellum are not connected, while those of the thalamocortical system are. A very simple observation in itself, but it is anything but trivial if one is equipped with a theory.

The cerebellum does not have a corpus callosum (Figure 6.1). The 35 billion neurons that inhabit the right hemisphere are completely separate from the 35 billion neurons in the left. A huge split-brain! This is not a good sign for integration and it immediately rings a warning bell. But, wait! Forty billion neurons are not to be sniffed at, after all they still are double the number of those present in the entire thalamocortical system. Why can't the two cerebellar hemispheres be superconscious twins? At this point, more butchering with our bare hands would not help; we need to borrow the neuro-anatomist's paraphernalia. To proceed with our investigations, we have to sit down and patiently examine how the neurons in each cerebellar hemisphere are interconnected.

If we were to do just that, we would conclude that the cerebellum is not only devoid of a corpus callosum to connect the two hemispheres, but that there are no long-range reciprocal connections within the different

CEREBELLUM

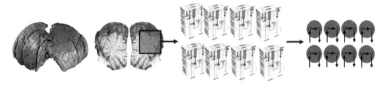

THALAMOCORTICAL SYSTEM

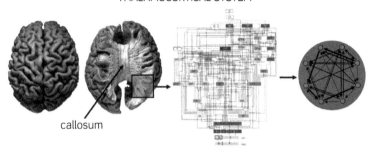

callosum

Figure 6.1 A comparison between the architecture of the cerebellum (top) and the one of the thalamocortical system (bottom). (Top left) Opening between the two hemispheres of the cerebellum, reveals the complete absence of connections between the right and the left side of the structure. (Bottom left) Instead, the two hemispheres of the cerebral cortex are connected by the 200 million fibers of the corpus callosum. (Top center) a microscopic examination shows that the cerebellar cortex is composed of myriads of segregated feed-forward circuits that do not form an integrated entity. (Bottom center) conversely, the cerebral cortex is characterized by a balanced architecture that is, at once, highly integrated and highly differentiated. This is exemplified here by the Van Essen Matrix, which summarizes the connectivity patterns of the visual system. (Top and bottom right) simplified models of the general architectures of the cerebellum and of the thalamocortical system.

zones of each cerebellar hemisphere. In essence, the cerebellum turns out to be composed of myriads of independent modules [153]. That is, it appears to be structured in such a way that once the signals reach the appropriate module, they remain confined there and do not influence other modules in any way. The electrical impulses enter each module of the cerebellum, are processed, and are quickly (within 10–20 ms) spat out by the other end of the circuit. As can be seen in Figure 6.1 (upper panel), the 70 billion neurons of the cerebellum are arranged in a series of segregated structures juxtaposed together, each of which receives and transmits signals that it does not share with the other modules.

This characteristic architecture of the cerebellum has been known for some time. It accounts for the extraordinary speed and precision with which this organ regulates movement and other functions. The set-up of the cerebellum resembles a series of small processors arranged in parallel lines, each of which carries out its specific task with remarkable precision and rapidity. Take movement, for example. Each module receives two forms of input. On the one hand, motor signals that provide instructions as to how a certain aspect of the movement is to be carried out; on the other hand, sensory information regarding the current state of affairs in the outside word. Each module compares the two signals, makes the appropriate calculations and emits instructions for any necessary adjustments to prevent errors. In this process, the cerebellar modules, which are extremely plastic, adapt to new conditions and learn to predict so that the adjustment signals become faster and increasingly more precise [154, 155]. This is how the cerebellum progressively assumes ownership of all motor patterns that initially have to be learned slowly, making a conscious effort. As a result, we are able to reach out a hand and grasp a glass of water without having to make conscious calculations of the weights and distances involved, or run our fingers over the keyboard of a piano to produce a harmonious sequence of notes without thinking. Seen from this point of view, this whole process is astounding. These modules deserve gratitude for their crystalline efficiency, flexibility, and the incredible speed with which they perform their tasks. For all this, the cerebellum pays a high price—it lacks integration. Even more, each cerebellar circuit seems to be organized in a series of feed-forward steps, with no recurrent excitation [156], an arrangement that is, as we shall see in Chapter 8, at least in principle, compatible with $\Phi = 0$.

We can hold the cerebellum in our hands as one object, it has one name and it owns one chapter in each textbook of physiology. Like the camera, it is considered to be a single entity. However, its unity is just an illusion, which disintegrates as soon as it is investigated correctly, with the appropriate rationale. Regardless of the immense quantity of neurons, synapses, and neurotransmitters; the richness of incoming and outgoing signals; its interconnections with the rest of the brain, including the cerebral cortex; notwithstanding all this, the cerebellum as such just does not exist. It is another example of ontological mistake, which is promptly revealed by Occam's razor in the form of Φ. What does exist is a vast number of individual modules, separate and free-standing, each with an information integration capacity that, if anything, is only slightly higher than that of a photodiode. Elegant and intricate as it may be, the cerebellum is not a unitary system with countless states at its disposal, but a collection of countless elements, each with just a few states to hand. For quite some time now, scientists and clinicians have known that what the cerebellum learns to do suddenly falls below the radar of consciousness and, when it is physically removed from the cranium, consciousness continues as before. Now we are perhaps closer to understanding why this is so.

It is time to turn our attention to the thalamocortical system. There can be no doubt that the presence of the corpus callosum bodes well for integration, but it is not an essential condition. Even if the neurosurgeon cuts with his knife the 200 million fibers of the callosum, each hemisphere is still able to generate its own consciousness, albeit perhaps with a somewhat diminished repertoire. So, once again, we will have to arm ourselves with the appropriate finer methodology to examine the intricate forest of neurons and connections, in the cerebral cortex this time. In addition to the corpus callosum, the thalamocortical system has bundles of short- and long-distance fibers, some of which connect directly neurons that are far apart (Figure 6.1, lower panel). These fibers criss-cross each hemisphere from top to bottom, from side to side and diagonally, tracing straight lines, wide arcs, and narrow curves. In appearance, they resemble a road map, with "speedways" connecting the neural groups of various cortical lobes, with millions of minor roads branching off from them, heading in all directions. The electrical impulses fly along these speedways, frequently in both directions, and then veer off onto motorways, then highways, local roads, lanes, even onto tiny alleys. This network is by no means homogeneous; the cerebral cortex hosts various neural "ethnic" groups, each with its own language, specificity, its particular set of connections, and preferences.

A "Holy Grail" of neuroscience is to figure out exactly how this neural melting pot is organized. The Human Genome Project that sequenced and mapped the genes of *Homo sapiens* was completed in 2003, after which the even more ambitious Human Connectome Project was launched in July 2009 [157]; top research centers and universities joined forces with the final goal of drawing a wiring diagram of the brain. A daunting proposition! To give an idea of the complexity of the project, the reconstruction of the brain of *Caenorhabditis elegans* (which despite the somewhat pretentious name is a free-living transparent roundworm about 1 mm in length), took about 12 years and was considered to be an exceptional feat [158]. However, the worm's brain is composed of only 302 neurons connected by 8000 synapses, whereas the numbers of the human brain connectome are simply breath-taking; billions of neurons, millions of miles of nerve fibers, and many more connections than the genome has letters. A square millimeter of cerebral cortex, which would be comparable to the volume of the entire *C. elegans*, contains approximately 150,000 neurons, each of which receives something like 10,000 synapses. This gives an idea of the immensity of the task that the Connectome Project is undertaking.

Despite of this level of complexity, some general principles of the architecture of the human thalamocortical system have been understood well enough to enable us to draw two important conclusions. The first is that the structure of this system is characterized by an exquisite degree of functional specialization [159]. Cortical neurons are connected to each other in such a way that each neuron tends to send and receive inputs and outputs to a distinct set of neighbors. As a consequence, each neuron is functionally specialized to respond to different inputs. In sensory regions in the back of the brain, this is reflected in the functional segregation between different areas and within each area. Different neurons in lower visual cortices respond to activity at different locations in the visual field, within each location they selectively respond to specific input features (such as orientation, spatial frequency, or wavelength). In higher areas, neurons respond to specific conjunctions of features (such as faces). More generally, neurons in different cortical areas respond to different dimensions (such as color and motion) or sensory modalities (such as vision or touch). The second conclusion is that these highly specialized neurons are, nevertheless, highly integrated. Especially in the posterior cortex, connections within each area are organized in a grid-like manner[1] and across areas in a pyramid-like, convergent/divergent manner. This kind of architecture leads to a high level of systematic overlap in the connections among neurons, giving rise to a core network that "hangs together" tightly—in other words, it is functionally highly integrated. In contrast, networks in which neurons are organized into segregated modules, such as the cerebellum, or in which the connections are organized more randomly, with less overlap, as may be the case in some parts of prefrontal cortex, are much less integrated. Of course, we should keep in mind that we are just starting to characterize the precise architecture of the human cortex and its multiscale complexity (from microscopic synaptic contacts to macroscopic fiber bundles), which will require combining atlases [160–162] and large-scale simulations [163–166]. Nevertheless, it seems fair to say that the thalamocortical system contains a structural core characterized by an effective combination of specialization and integration [167, 168]. Such a balanced anatomy is a necessary prerequisite to integrate information and suits well the empirical data highlighting the importance of the thalamocortical system for consciousness.

Going back to the theory, what are the implications of this brief analysis? The structural balance described above implies that, in the thalamocortical system, the activity of each neural group depends, and depends very specifically, on the activity of all the other groups. This means that the system as a whole can count on virtually infinite activity patterns. Going back to the light–dark experiment, it is evident that, in the thalamocortical system, darkness is darkness because the underlying activity pattern of cortical neurons is one out of an extraordinarily large number of alternative patterns, which would have been triggered by light, color, objects, sounds, feeling, and thoughts of all kinds. Every conscious experience corresponds to a unique shape that differs in its own specific way from all the other possible shapes, which as we have seen, are countless.

---

1 For an interesting discussion on whether and how grid-like architectures, such as the maps in visual cortex, may contribute to high level of information integration and to consciousness see https://www.scottaaronson.com/blog/?p=1823.

In this enormous framework, silent neurons are just as important as those that fire, just as the pauses in the music executed by great philharmonic orchestras count just as much, if not even more, than the actual notes played. How would we know that darkness is darkness and not blue, for example, without the possibility of having silent "blue" neurons? If the millions of modules that constitute our cerebral cortex were to be removed, one by one, leaving just the module that responds to "darkness," what would we see? Initially, darkness would not be distinguishable from blue, from an object, a face, or a sound, and at the end it would not be distinguishable from anything at all. In fact, darkness would be nothing. We would see nothing and be nothing. Even if the darkness module, in total isolation, were still able to command the muscles of the mouth to say "darkness," the word would have no meaning; it would be a word without consciousness.

Figure 6.2 illustrates a notable clinical correlate of this principle. Nikolas Schiff of the University of New York studied a group of VS/UWS patients, all of whom had retained only very small islands of cortical matter following severe brain injuries [169]. One patient in particular presented an interesting case; in her devastated brain, a few modules belonging to the language area had remained alive—they could still receive auditory inputs and control some muscles to utter words in Spanish and English. These words, however, were produced at random and made no sense, being spoken out of context. Indeed, the patient had been in a VS/UWS for over 20 years following a lesion that destroyed most of the cortex. Those pronounced by a group of survivor neurons isolated from the loom of the thalamocortical system were certainly words, but words without mind.

This clinical example underscores a crucial point that is often forgotten. It is commonly assumed loosely that the firing of specific cortical neurons, e.g., those for black, conveys some specific information, e.g., that there is something black, and that such information becomes conscious either as such or perhaps if it is disseminated widely. However, if one thinks carefully, a given cortical element has no information about whether what made it fire was a particular color, rather than a face, a visual stimulus rather than a sound, a sensory stimulus, rather than a thought. All it knows is whether it fired or not, just as each receiving element only knows whether it received an input or not. Thus, the information specifying "black" cannot possibly be in the message conveyed

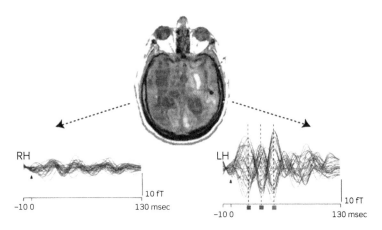

RH

LH

10 fT
−10 0   130 msec

10 fT
−10 0   130 msec

Figure 6.2 Words without mind. A woman, unconscious for 20 years, spontaneously produces infrequent, isolated words unrelated to any environmental context. The yellow areas depicted on the brain indicate small cortical territories with preserved metabolism (as measured with PET) in the left hemisphere. Below, magnetoencephalographic (MEG) recordings are shown, identifying patterns of evoked brain activity in response to auditory stimulation only in the left hemisphere (LH). The observation demonstrates that isolated neuronal groups may express well-defined fragments of activity in a severely damaged, unconscious brain.

Reproduced from Nicholas Schiff, Urs Ribary, Fred Plum and Rodolfo Llinás, Words without mind, *Journal of Cognitive Neuroscience*, 6(11), pp. 650–6, doi: 10.1162/089892999563715. © 1999, Massachusetts Institute of Technology. Reprinted by permission of MIT Press Journals.

by the firing of any neural element, whether it is located in a high-order cortical area or it is broadcasted globally. Crucially, according to IIT, that information is not in an extrinsic message, but resides instead in a form specified intrinsically by the system as a whole. This is an essential difference. For example, according to functionalistic, information-processing approaches, such as Global Workspace Theory, consciousness requires the active "broadcasting" of information. By contrast, IIT makes the highly counterintuitive neurophysiological prediction that consciousness should be present even when most neurons comprising the substrate of consciousness are inactive. What would it feel like? Perhaps, like the "pure consciousness" state or "core experience" documented over many centuries, and within many different cultural contexts and spiritual traditions—literally, an empty unity from which all multiplicities of sensuous, conceptual, or other empirical contents has been excluded [170].

Mystical experiences aside, this is where the thalamocortical system plays its ace, leaving astonished and confused philosophers, scientists, and laymen alike. When we see darkness, we think we are seeing darkness, that darkness exists out there, but this is far from the truth. The darkness that we see, that we imagine, that we dream of, exists only in relation to what could have been, but was not, to an immense repertoire of potential states. The form of darkness, with its uniqueness and richness, is woven on a perfectly balanced enchanted loom, in a split second and in one sole place where, at any given time, everything counts and where so much is possible. In this respect, the thalamocortical system is very different from the cerebellum and probably from any other object that we know of.

Other Mysteries Inside the Brain

Under the lens of IIT, the cerebellum disintegrated into a heap of dust, whereas from the thalamocortical system arose a majestic cathedral. Can something be said about other structures and paradoxes that lurk in the cranium?

The Retina and Sensory Systems

What we see normally depends on the pattern of electrical impulses that run across a neural pathway, which leads from the retina to the visual modules of the cerebral cortex. That said, the retina and the optic nerve do not contribute directly to conscious visual experience [133]. For example, we know that sudden changes in the activity of the retinal cells that occur during blinking and saccadic movements do not interfere with the stability of the image we perceive. We also know that there is a blind spot on the retina that is devoid of receptors, as well a peripheral portion of the retina that has a low spatial resolution and is not very sensitive to color. Yet, none of this affects our conscious visual experience— we are not aware of the blind spot, and we do not see a pixelated, black and white peripheral visual field. Not to mention that acquired retinal blindness does not prevent us from imagining colorful, vivid scenes, and that whatever we dream visually has nothing to do with the neural impulses running in the optic nerve. To sum up, it is clear that while the retina and the optic nerve help us to see what is in the world around us, they are neither necessary nor are they sufficient in themselves to generate a conscious visual experience in any given moment. All this is well known, but deserves an explanation.

Let's see whether a theoretical principle can help. Take a small model of the thalamocortical system, which includes a tiny retina, that is a number of parallel incoming neural chains. If we measure Φ for this group of elements, we will immediately identify the weak link. There is a partition of this system across which little information is integrated, much less than that integrated by one of its parts (Figure 6.3A). This particular cut excludes the incoming retinal chain and shows that the system as a whole integrates less information than the eight-element complex that replicates the general architecture of the thalamocortical system.

Going back to the real brain, it is useful to recall that light and dark only exist in relation to the immense number of possibilities available to a system that is at once integrated and differentiated. The retina and the optic fibers are characterized by a segregated architecture that is very similar to that which characterizes the sensor of the camera and the modules of the cerebellum, and so do not take part to the core with maximum Φ. This way visual afferent neurons, like all the other sensory pathways that run parallel towards the cerebral cortex, can influence the firing of the thalamocortical neurons without in any way influencing its capacity for integrating information. The hard core of the thalamocortical system, with its vast repertoire of causal relations, can be influenced in what it sees and hears via the sense organs, but it can also see and hear without them. For this reason, we can imagine and dream with our eyes shut.

Motor Systems

What we have just said about sensory pathways also applies to motor outputs. We tend to associate the presence of consciousness with the observation of a repertoire of gestures and purposeful movements, both in everyday life and in clinical neurological practice. If we ask a person a number of questions and receive specific responses to each, then we assume that the person is conscious. This criterion is quite reasonable from the point of view of integrated information, given that a wide range

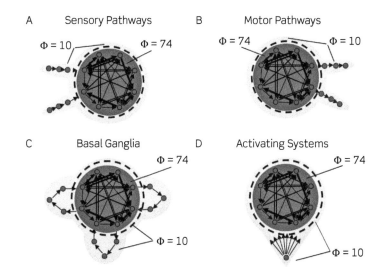

Figure 6.3 Four simplified models illustrate the general architecture of (A) the sensory pathways, (B) the motor pathways, (C) the basal ganglia, (D) the activating systems, and the corresponding values of integrated information. The blue dots represent the elements (neurons) and the arrows the connections between them. For each model, the grey dark area represents the partition of the system with maximum Φ. The light grey area indicates the larger system with lower Φ and the dotted lines highlight the weak links.

of behaviors indicates that the integrated system has a vast repertoire of available states at its disposal. This notwithstanding, the neural activity of the motor system does not appear to be a necessary condition for being conscious. As we saw earlier in this book, patients suffering from LIS are fully conscious, even though they are almost completely paralyzed [47]. This is also true for whoever dreams during REM sleep, when motor outputs are actively inhibited by physiological mechanisms [80]. Why do motor outputs not contribute directly to conscious experience, even though they are essential for behaviors that express the rich conscious life going on inside the skull? As with sensory input from the retina, and as illustrated in Figure 6.3B, efferent motor pathways, running in parallel, like those of the senses, are not included in the complex with high Φ.

Basal Ganglia

As mentioned in Chapter 2, besides the cerebellum, there is another major zombie in the brain, the basal ganglia. These are large structures, located just below the cortex, capable of producing highly complicated behaviors. However, once again, the neural processes that take place in these subcortical nuclei do not seem necessary for consciousness. Although the basal ganglia are crucial in maintaining the excitability of frontal executive and motor circuits [141], it is known that large, hemorrhagic lesions can occur without significant alteration in the level of consciousness [171]. For example, children affected by familial bilateral basal ganglia necrosis may not be able to speak, but are able to respond to sensory stimuli and communicate with their parents in other ways [142]. Similarly, adults with late onset familial dystonia and lesions throughout the basal ganglia may develop cognitive problems, which can include a frontal syndrome, but are nonetheless clearly conscious [143].The basal ganglia are inserted into various circuits, some of which involved in the production of language, others in controlling movement, others deal with the cognitive functions, others with social behaviors, motivation, and the regulation of emotion. Each circuit originates from a specific module in the cerebral cortex, passes through the basal ganglia via the thalamus, then returns to the cortex. From an anatomical point of view, the basal ganglia appear as a group of parallel, feed-forward neural chains [172, 173]. How is it possible that such complex structures, so closely associated to thalamocortical circuits and capable of influencing its functioning, do not contribute to consciousness? As illustrated in Figure 6.3C, parallel loops can be informationally excluded by the main complex, even though they are connected to it by both input and output sides. This is interesting as it suggests that some subcortical cycles or loops may implement specialized subroutines that are capable of influencing the states of the main corticothalamic complex without joining it. Such informationally insulated cortico-subcortical-cortical loops could constitute the neural substrates for many unconscious processes that can affect and be affected by conscious experience. Metaphorically speaking, the cortical modules are located in the control room, where all the important decisions are taken in a consensus meeting, whereas subcortical loops represent a sort of private line for technical data processing, for the use of individual cortical elements. Together with the cerebellum, the basal ganglia circuits supply uninterrupted unconscious support to our conscious life. When we speak aloud, or talk to ourselves in our head, when we type on a keyboard or write with a pen, automatic routines and subroutines are continuously at work to find the right word, to check our grammar, and transmit the results to our consciousness for the next iteration. The support of unconscious routines to our conscious existence is always there: not only when we speak, write, play a musical instrument or engage in physical activities—it is also present when we are involved in purely cognitive tasks, such as when we calculate, when we think, and when we make plans. Many thought sequences and associations are automatic and take place without our being aware of the processes behind them, for better or for worse. They are, to all extents and purposes, beyond our control. Just imagine millions of feed-forward rings placed in parallel rows, receiving and re-transmitting sequences of impulses to the conscious parts of the thalamocortical complex, sequences that will be modified, adjusted, and sometimes even distorted depending on experience and habit.

At this point, the question arises as to what is the share of total brain activity that does not directly contribute to experience. If we consider the amount of activity of the segregated modules of the cerebellum and that carried out in the millions of loops that constitute the basal ganglia, then it is reasonable to suppose that a substantial part of what the neurons do remains in the realm of the unconscious. In these terms, IIT also accounts for the vastness of the unconscious and the unpredictable conditioning that it exerts on our everyday life.

Activating Systems

Lesions of the activating systems of the brainstem may cause loss of consciousness and coma (see Chapter 3). Conversely, as the physiologists Moruzzi and Magoun demonstrated in 1949, electrical stimulation of these neural systems can provoke widespread activation of the thalamocortical system and bring an animal out of a comatose state [144]. The neural groups that compose the activating systems release a family of neuromodulators such as acetylcholine, histamine, noradrenaline, serotonin, dopamine, and glutamate, which can regulate the excitability of the entire thalamocortical system [174]. Basically, they function as a switch, impacting the general state of the system. However, activating systems do not appear to make a specific contribution to experience and, most important, they are not sufficient for consciousness, as we have seen in VS/UWS patients. Why is this so?

Figure 6.3D provides a schematic representation of how the activating systems are arranged anatomically, showing a single element that project diverging inputs to all thalamocortical elements. Although the activating element is connected to each and every element of a system with high Φ, it remains excluded from it. From the standpoint of information integration, the activating system neuron and the eight thalamocortical neurons do, indeed, form a system, but one with a lower Φ. Again, IIT's Occam's razor eliminates everything that is not strictly necessary and suggests that if we were to find a direct way of effectively activating thalamocortical neurons, whether with direct electric neuromodulation or chemically, it might be possible to restore consciousness to a patient whose brainstem switch has been irreparably broken.

The Split-Brain

Consciousness divides when the corpus callosum is severed. Surprisingly, neither the level nor the content of the consciousness of the dominating hemisphere are significantly modified by this operation and even the non-dominant hemisphere, while losing some important abilities, such as speech, continues to host a conscious individual. What can IIT say about this phenomenon? Clearly, the 200 million fibers that connect the two hemispheres bidirectionally are sufficient to ensure that the thalamocortical system taken as a whole integrates more information than the hemispheres would on their own, which is why each of us is a single conscious being, not two. By the same token, when the corpus callosum is severed, the two hemispheres cannot form a single integrated complex, and consciousness splits, exactly as one would expect if consciousness requires information integration [145, 151]. On the other hand, because the two hemispheres are organized quite similarly, except for a few functions, such as language, there is a fair amount of redundancy in their information capacity, because much of the states that are intrinsically available to the left are duplicated in the right. So, the prediction of

IIT is that the value of Φ of each hemisphere in the split-brain condition should not be dramatically less or dramatically different to when the two hemispheres are united. Moreover, IIT makes an intriguing prediction, because what matters is always the maximum of integrated information, if we were to cut the callosum progressively, axon-by-axon, there would be a singularity; a precise moment where the two hemisphere would become two maxima with Φ values higher than that value for the whole brain. At that precise moment, one consciousness would split in two.

Time and Consciousness

Conscious experience requires a special architecture, but time as well [175, 176]. For example, in order to elicit a conscious sensation by means of direct cortical stimulation in humans the train of electrical pulses must last for about 500 ms and evoked activations of shorter duration generally fail to yield a subjective report [177]. Along the same lines, psychophysiological studies have demonstrated that it can take up to 200–300 ms to attain the full perception of a sensory stimulus [178]. Thus, entering a given conscious state seems to require a minimal duration of neural activity that amounts to few hundred milliseconds. Of course, the brain can detect relevant stimuli and supply useful responses quicker than this, but these are not conscious reactions. When we touch a burning hot surface and our hand snaps away in a reflex action, or when an athlete springs off blocks 120 ms after the "bang" of the starter's gun, there is no doubt that the stimulus has been somehow processed by neural circuits, but the experience of the pain of the burn, or the sound of the starter's gun, comes after. The emergence of a visual percept is rather like the development of a film and unfolds on the time scale of a few hundred milliseconds: first, we are aware something has happened, then we become aware of the "gist" of a scene, telling us that we are outdoors, rather than indoors, then elementary characteristics, such as movement, appear, the spatial orientation, the approximate dimensions, and then forms and colors, followed by the formation of various objects and our recognition of them as such. Why is this so?

According to IIT, even the simple experience of darkness corresponds to a unique shape that is specified by distributed causal interactions within the thalamocortical system. If darkness is to be darkness and not light, or blue, or a face, or a sound or a taste, if it is to have meaning for us, neurons located far apart need to affect each other to build up a specific pattern of activity. Inevitably, in the wet matter of the brain this process takes time.

Neurons have certain biophysical characteristics, including finite conduction velocities and relatively slow impulse response properties. In practice, neural impulses travel along the axons at a rate that depends on the caliber of the axon and its degree of insulation. The most rapid travels at the equivalent of 50 m/s, around 180 km/h, but some fibers do not support such speed, and the impulse will not reach more than 0.3 m/s, just a little over 1 km/h. Fortunately, the distances in the brain are measured in centimeters and not in kilometers, so the time it takes to travel from point A to point B is just a fraction of a second, say 10–100 ms depending on the destination and on how well the axon is insulated. Once the impulse has arrived at destination, it has to be transmitted from neuron A to neuron B, which takes more time, partly due to synaptic delays and partly (the lion's share) to the time required for neuron B to build up a supra-threshold response and fire an impulse. This last step is the most critical because neuron B may emit an impulse only if it integrates many inputs coming from neuron A and other neurons, which can take from just a few milliseconds to tens of milliseconds. Scaling up the example, it is clear that building-up a chain of reliable and specific causal interactions among distributed groups of neurons, takes some time. After a few milliseconds, causal interactions would be zero and the system would be totally disintegrated, after a few tens of milliseconds, causal interactions would start to become effective, but they would still be unreliable and poorly differentiated, only later they would stabilize in a specific form, thanks to both feed-forward and feed-back connection, to finally dissipate back into the sea of spontaneous brain activity. In essence, there is an optimal time interval at which the brain makes more difference to itself. It is important to remark that, according to IIT, the delay of experience is not due to the time it takes for an extrinsic piece of information to travel and be broadcast in the brain, but to the time the physical brain takes to create information, from its intrinsic perspective. Crucially, the optimal timescale at which Φ reaches a maximum should be consistent with estimates of the time scale of experience. Based on what we know from phenomenology, the instant of consciousness is definite, ranging from a several tens of milliseconds to a few hundred milliseconds, rather than lasting a few milliseconds or a few seconds [146]. This is a well-known, non-trivial fact for which IIT tries to provide a principled explanation.

Now, it is also somewhat easier to understand why the cerebellum and the basal ganglia are so much quicker than we consciously are. These zombies, so useful and swift, do not integrate information and all the neural processes remain segregated in local feed-forward circuits with a much faster time constant. We, as conscious beings, are much slower and much clumsier, but this is the price we have to pay for building up an intrinsic perspective. All-in-all, it is a price we pay willingly, because we are all in the same boat and because we have the suspicion that time itself would not exist if experience was not there to mark it.

CHAPTER 7

ASSESSING CONSCIOUSNESS IN OTHER HUMANS: FROM THEORY TO PRACTICE

Looking at neuroanatomy through the lens of a theory has provided useful insights and plausible explanations for fundamental observations, as well as puzzling paradoxes. We tried to find our way through a tangle of billions of neurons and emerged with some criteria that allowed us to recognize certain complicated brain structures that are, nevertheless, unsuited to integrating information—such as the cerebellum and the basal ganglia—and thus cannot support consciousness, but only "zombie" systems. Now it's time to move on and ask what changes when consciousness fades during sleep and anesthesia, or recovers during a dream, even though the structure of the brain remains the same. Most important, in doing so, we would like to improve our ability to detect consciousness at the bedside of patients, irrespective of sensory processing and responsiveness, based on the guidelines provided by IIT. If consciousness depends on the brain's capacity to integrate information, we must find practical ways to measure it. Galileo said: "Measure what can be measured, and make measurable what cannot be measured." We need to build a new kind of telescope, one that is perhaps very primitive, but that is designed according to first principles.

Difficult to Achieve, Difficult to Measure

It is now obvious that measuring levels of neural activity will not be sufficient to obtain even the roughest estimate of Φ. In fact, just as integrated information is not determined by the number of elements in a system (as illustrated by the model in the bottom panel of Figure 5.3 and by the para-digmatic case of the cerebellum), it is not necessarily affected by the overall amount of neuronal firing. To the extreme, if all cortical neurons fired at their maximum capacity, but their synaptic connections were disabled, Φ would be zero because the brain would lack intrinsic cause–effect power.

Empirical measures designed to capture the synergy among distant groups of neurons are certainly more interesting in this context. As briefly outlined in Chapter 3, these indices rely on the principle of temporal cor-relation, that is on the assumption that groups of neurons, which show activity patterns that are coordinated it time, are also linked by reciprocal causal interactions. However, this is not necessarily true. In fact, there can be cases in which high levels of synchrony are achieved among elements that are actually segregated. All it takes is a common driver, a hidden neur-onal source that imposes its own activity pattern through feed-forward connections to all the other elements. In this master-and-slave arrange-ment, such as the one illustrated in Figure 6.3D, all receiving neurons can display high levels of temporal correlation even in the complete absence of reciprocal causal interactions. In such cases, one would be inclined to infer integration where there is none, which is to commit the fatal ontological error of taking an aggregate of independent elements for a unity. There is plenty of room for such a misunderstanding in the realm of neurophysi-ology, because there are many common drivers, from correlated sensory inputs to neuronal pace-makers hidden in the depth of the brain.

An additional problem with measures of temporal correlation is that high synchrony among distant group neurons implies that different elements are engaged in similar patterns of activity, which corresponds to a decrease of overall differentiation within the system. In practice, the more we try to be sensitive to neural integration by classic indices of temporal correlation, the more we miss the information part of the story. Now, it may not come as a surprise that, in some conditions, such as during a seizure, indices of synchrony peak as consciousness fades. When integration is maximal, information can be minimal, which may explain why measures of synchrony do not discriminate reliably at the single-subject level between consciousness and unconsciousness.

Clearly, information must also be seriously taken into account and measured explicitly. The simplest way to quantify information from brain signals is measuring their variability or entropy. This principle is widely applied to neural activity in more or less formal ways. For example, neurologists typically look to the differentiation of EEG rhythms, their reactivity, and tendency to change in time and space, whereas anesthesiologists have been building simple machines that record brain activity in the operating room and output entropy-related empirical indices of the level of consciousness, such as the bi-spectral index [179]. The general assumption is that a conscious brain that receives and processes different stimuli shows more variable patterns with higher entropy. One problem with this approach is that entropy-related measures reach maximal values for random signals, which is for patterns that can be produced by noisy systems that are everything, but complex and interesting. However, the key issue is that entropy per se is not sensitive to whether the information it quantifies is generated by one single system or by a collection of many. Taking this argument to the extreme, the entropy of a disconnected cortex, where isolated elements run freely according to their own pace, would be maximal, just like the entropy generated by the 1 million independent photodiodes seizing with static noise. This lack of sensitivity for causality and integration is probably one of the reasons why current indices of information are not up to the task when it comes to reliably assessing consciousness in the brain of individual subjects [180].

In essence, besides the technical difficulties inherent to detecting genuine integration and information per se, there is a more general issue—empirical indices that are sensitive to integration have low sensitivity to information, whereas measures that are sensitive to information have low sensitivity to integration. The coexistence of unity and diversity is not only difficult to achieve in physical systems, but also difficult to measure. This is a non-trivial task [181, 182], which requires thinking, effort, and a precise theoretical motivation.

Assessing Integrated Information: From Theory to Practice

The principle outlined in Chapter 5 provides the rationale to guide the design of such a novel measurement tool. According to IIT, what we need to gauge is the amount of information that is generated through causal interactions within the brain. With this in mind, we can list a few practical rules:

Rule 1: Observing is not enough, one needs to perturb and detect cause–effect relationships. As we have already discussed, neurons that are segregated may show synchronous activity simply because they receive common inputs. To unmask this false integration one can resort to perturbations, that is, stimulate directly a subset of neurons and measure the effects of their activation on the rest of the brain. In the presence of genuine integration, the initial activation will trigger a chain of widespread cause–effect interactions across the system. Otherwise, the effects of the perturbation will remain local, irrespective of the observable level of synchrony.

Rule 2: Detecting widespread responses is not enough; one needs to assess their differentiation. Making sure that the system is one is a key step, but it is not sufficient. A large integrated system that is only capable of global, all-or-nothing responses, such as a huge photodiode or the beating heart, is not a suitable physical substrate of consciousness. Clearly, one needs to check to what extent the cause–effect mechanisms within the system are differentiated. This can be done by assessing the complexity of the effects of the perturbation. Only in a brain that is, at once, integrated and differentiated, will the perturbation engage many distributed elements in specific ways, resulting in a rich spatiotemporal dynamics that is complex and difficult to describe.

Rule 3: Responses must be recorded on an adequate time scale. As we know from phenomenology, consciousness has a definite time scale, ranging from tens of milliseconds to a few hundred milliseconds. Thus, the relevant cause–effect interactions must occur with a similar temporal grain. This requires recording the brain's response to the perturbation with a sub-second time resolution.

Rule 4: The measurement must bypass sensory inputs and motor outputs. In Chapter 5, "A Theoretical Principle," we have seen that parallel incoming and outgoing neural chains are not part of the main complex as these channels represent weak links. Likewise, we have considered practical cases in which consciousness may be present, but not accessible from the outside world just because afferent and efferent pathways are blocked or disabled. Thus, it is fundamental to directly probe the core of the thalamocortical system independently of sensory processing and motor behavior.

A summary of these four guidelines can be formulated as:

> Evaluating a brain's capacity to integrate information requires direct perturbations of cortical neurons (bypass input and output chains) to assess the spatial extent of the evoked response (integration) and its differentiation (information content) on a sub-second time scale (time constant of consciousness).

Putting this in layman's terms, we need to find ways to directly perturb the thalamocortical complex and listen to the echo it produces [183], a way of proceeding very similar to what we would do with any unknown object; we knock on it with our knuckles and deduce what it might contain based on the sound it makes. If the theoretical postulates are correct, a conscious brain should sound very different from an unconscious one, as schematically illustrated in Figure 7.1. When consciousness is lost, the echo will either be local, because only the subset of elements that are directly perturbed and not more distant elements, will respond to the stimulation (low integration), or it will be global, but stereotypical, because all elements will respond in the same way (low information). The echo will be both global and differentiated, that is complex, only if many elements interact through specific mechanisms (integrated information).

Of course, characterizing this echo is still a far cry from calculating Φ, which would require perturbing the brain in all possible ways across all possible bipartitions [147, 149]. Yet, this approach is directly inspired by phenomenological principles and it offers, for the first time, a viable way to jointly gauge unity and difference, causality and information directly in the black box of the brain.

A Magnetic Probe to Appreciate the Echo of Consciousness

Before putting principles into practice, there are technical issues to be solved. The central challenge is to find a way of directly activating a subset of cortical neurons, and recording the response of the rest of the brain with good spatial and temporal resolution. Of course, this needs to be done non-invasively (without sticking electrodes inside the brain) and possibly at the bedside of the patient. Fortunately, it turns out that all this can be done without inventing radically new machines; the innovation is to be found in the concept, rather than in the means. A radically new strategy of measurement can be obtained using two old instruments, magnetic brain stimulation and EEG, both of which have almost a century of honored service to their merit.

The history of magnetic stimulation dates back to the dawn of the 1900s, from the stories of the strange experiences recounted by workers in the first power stations. They told of bizarre and inexplicable sensations, hallucinations, intermittent glows, and sudden shafts of light. It was not long before it was realized that these strange phenomena were not casual, but occurred when the men were working in the neighborhood of the great copper bobbins with the high tension current. Silvanus Phillips Thompson, a Fellow of the Royal Society, investigated the phenomenon in 1910, developing the first rudimentary transcranial magnetic stimulator (TMS; Figure 7.2A). The instrument was made of two large coils of copper wire, and the patient was seated with his head between the two coils. A strong electrical current (approximately 180 Amps) was then passed through the coils. Those who were brave enough to undertake the treatment reported hallucinations, unexpected bursts of light in various areas of their visual field, and a strange after-taste on the tongue. These sensory effects were caused by magnetic induction as described by Michael Faraday more than half a century earlier; the electric current that ran through the copper wire coiled into the bobbins generated a magnetic field that penetrated skin and bone, reaching and stimulating the neurons to generate electrical impulses, which the brain interpreted as light and taste. At the time, the question as to whether the strange effects reported by subjects were due to a stimulation of the peripheral nerves or to a direct effect on cortical neurons was to remain unanswered. The world had to wait until 1985, when Anthony Barker of the University of Sheffield tried out the first modern TMS on the head of one of his collaborators [184]. He positioned his instrument correspondingly with the area of the cerebral cortex that commands hand movements and threw the switch, releasing a tension of approximately 10,000 V into the bobbins. After about 10 ms the collaborator's hand jerked, just like the hand of a puppet manipulated by his master. TMS generated a strong (1–2 T) and brief (0.3 ms) magnetic field, which induced an electric field sufficient to elicit a burst of action potentials in a subset of cortical neurons. The electrical impulses ran down the axons towards the spinal cord and the peripheral nerves, eliciting a muscle contraction. From that day on, TMS became the primary instrument for studying the state of motor cortex and of the neural fibers running down to muscles.

The possibility of directly stimulating a selected subset of cortical neurons through the scalp is an excellent starting point for approximating the theoretical measurement we have in mind. However, we are not interested in how neural activity moves along motor fibers, which has nothing to do with consciousness; we want to record the echo that the magnetic perturbation produces in the whole thalamocortical system. In fact, rather more than that; we want to know if and how the echo changes when consciousness disappears and when it recovers. This is where another veteran of the neurophysiological arsenal comes to our aid: the EEG (Figure 7.2B).

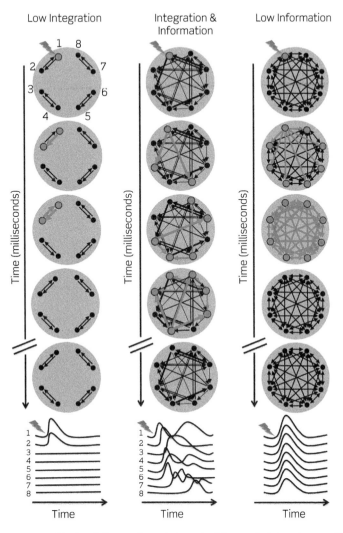

Figure 7.1 An idealized illustration of the principles underlying the empirical approximation of Φ. The same simplified models of eight elements described in Figure 5.3 are considered. The jagged red arrow indicates the perturbation; active elements and connections are depicted in red. The traces at the bottom represent the time-course of activity recorded from each element within the systems. Left column: low integration; perturbing the first element results in a short-leaved, local activation involving only the element connected to the perturbed one. Right

The idea is very simple, at least on paper: first knock on the cerebral cortex with TMS and then listen to the brain's echo with the EEG. TMS turns on a group of cortical neurons, which react by generating electrical impulses impacting upon other cortical neurons and so on, finally triggering a chain reaction that resonates within the entire system. By applying a large number of electrodes to the patient's scalp and connecting them to a special TMS-compatible EEG amplifier, it is possible to pick up the echo of the rush of electrical activation throughout the brain, with millisecond precision [185]. The more the brain is integrated and differentiated, the more global and complex will be the causal chain of electrical events triggered by TMS. At last, we have the necessary equipment for our investigations: a rudimentary electromagnetic telescope to glimpse at the physical substrate of consciousness, which we will henceforth call TMS/EEG (Figure 7.2C). Now theory can be translated into practice:

> TMS can be used to stimulate a subset of cortical neurons (direct access to the main complex) and the EEG to record the extension (integration) and the complexity (information) of the electrical response produced by the thalamocortical system on a sub-second time scale (time constant of consciousness).

Having described the basic approach and the experimental set-up, we now ask the reader to join us in the laboratory to get a practical feel of the data we can acquire with TMS/EEG. In the following, there will be a slight change of tone; we will try to summarize almost 15 years of trial and error, sleepless nights, technical mishaps, and above all, of passionate team work distributed between the University of Wisconsin, the ComaScience Group at the University of Liege, and the University of Milan. Here, nostalgic shades and occasional bursts of enthusiasm will be unavoidable, but let's state clearly the hypothesis to be tested—the

---

column: low information; perturbing the first element results in a widespread, all-or-none activation. Central column: integrated information; only in this case, perturbing the first element results in a widespread, complex response involving different elements at different time intervals.

Reproduced from Simone Sarasso, Mario Rosanova, Adenauer G. Casali, Silvia Casarotto, Matteo Fecchio, Melanie Boly, Olivia Gosseries, Giulio Tononi, Steven Laureys, and Marcello Massimini, *Clinical EEG and Neuroscience*, 45(1), pp. 40–9, doi: 10.1177/1550059413513723, © 2014 SAGE Publications. Reprinted by permission of SAGE Publications, Inc.

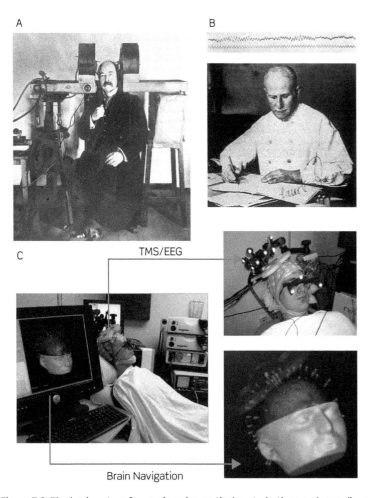

Figure 7.2 The basic set-up for non-invasive cortical perturbations and recordings. (A) The first transcranial magnetic stimulator, developed by Silvanus Phillips Thompson in the early 1900s. (B) One of the first systems for EEG recordings in humans, employed by Hans Berger in Germany in 1924. (C) The basic components of the TMS/EEG set-up used in the experiments described in this chapter. The subject wears a 60-channel EEG cap (blue) connected to a TMS-compatible EEG amplifier. The TMS coil is positioned at the desired location on the subject's head. Passive sensors (white spheres) mounted on the TMS coil and on the subject's head are tracked by an infrared camera and their relative position is co-registered with the individual subject's structural MRI. The monitor of the navigation system displays in

EEG response to TMS will be widespread and complex in a conscious brain and will be local (loss of integration), and/or less complex (loss of information) whenever consciousness fades.

Dreamless Sleep

Watching in real time the encephalogram of a person slipping into sleep is an absorbing and fascinating experience. It is like contemplating a fireplace or the ocean. The traces of electrical activity picked up by dozens of EEG sensors appear on the monitor as bursts of flames, licking the darkness with tongues of light, or caressing it like the waves on the shore. You could watch it for hours, mesmerized. When the person enters deep sleep, the sea whips up into a tempest; the myriad rivulets of the waking hours swirl into huge waves of electric activity, sometimes slow and majestic, at other times capped with white horses, small, sharp fluctuations that seem to be created by sudden gusts of wind. The brain seems to be more agitated in the sleeping state than when it is awake, but the level of consciousness dwindles until it disappears altogether. Why is this? It is now clear that addressing this question requires more than just an observation of the surface. We have to toss a stone into the water.

The first TMS/EEG measurement at the boundary of consciousness came after 1 year of testing and fine tuning of equipment and procedures. Finally, we enlisted our first subject, a young student from the Department of Philosophy at the University of Wisconsin. We explained to him once more what the experiment consisted of, while we applied 60 electrodes to his head. Then we showed him the probe, which is to all effects and purposes a 10-cm wide magnet, and explained that we would use this device to briefly activate a 2-cm² patch of neurons in his cerebral cortex. We told him that he wouldn't feel a thing during the stimulation and that all he had

---

real-time a 3D reconstruction of the patient's brain, the position of the TMS and an estimation of the intensity of the electric field generated on the cortical surface. In this way, TMS can be targeted to specific cortical areas at the desired intensity of stimulation.

Figure 7.2a: Reproduced by permission of Archives Imperial College London. Figure 7.2b: Photo by Apic/Getty Images.

to do was relax in the comfortable reclining armchair. We told him that we were about to look into his brain as if we were technicians testing the circuits of a TV. We were just going to inject an electrical current at a specific point to see how it flowed into the elements of the system and what kind of effects it had. No task, no particular engagement, or behavior was requested on his side; he just had to try and fall asleep, although under these conditions this was not going to be easy, with dozens of cables attached to the head, unfamiliar machines studded with flickering LEDs, an infrared camera scrutinized him from its perch high in the ceiling, an image of his brain for him to see on the monitor, laid open without its skull, enveloped by a strange hood clustered with sensors, and the stimulator looming over him, held by a mechanical arm. No big deal, like many university students, he was naturally sleep-deprived and happy to rest on a comfortable chair with people getting busy around him. He actually reported the relaxing feel of sitting in a barbershop, ready to be shaved.

When everything was ready we asked the student to stay awake and, using neuro-navigation, we targeted the TMS probe and set it to the right intensity to activate cortical neurons. We turned on the stimulator, which started pinging the cortex regularly—once every 2 s or so—and we took our place in front of the monitor to appreciate the brain's electrical echo (Figure 7.3). The first measurement met our expectations. The initial activity, triggered by the magnetic perturbation in the site immediately below the stimulator, shifted from one cortical area to another, reverberating for approximately 300 ms. The end result was a complex chain of causal interactions, in which many areas, distributed across the cortex, lit up and shut down in different ways, and at different times (Figure 7.3, upper panel). We declared ourselves satisfied—we had knocked on the waking brain and had recorded the distant echo of diversity in unity.

Then we turned off the lights and told the student to try to catch some sleep. After about 20 min we were ready to probe, for the first time, a brain caught in the large waves of deep NREM sleep. We switched on the TMS again and aimed it at the coordinates of the same group of neurons that we had stimulated before, releasing the exact same magnetic field. We stared at the computer monitor glooming in the dark and after a few pulses of TMS the response of the sleeping brain was already clearly visible. The area just below the stimulator bounced with a positive–negative wave of electrical activity, which was obviously larger than the response recorded in wakefulness. However, the electrical symphony had gone!

It was almost as if the coarse physical composition of the brain had changed: the multiform echo that resounded through the entire cranium had given way to a dull thud [186]. The initial response was large, but did not propagate beyond the area that was being directly stimulated and the cerebral cortex seemed fragmented (Figure 7.3, lower panel). We shook the student awake and asked him what he was feeling, what he remembered of what was going on in his mind. The response? A laconic "Nothing," as if he had not been there.

Thus, below the agitated waves of spontaneous activity and their apparent synchrony, TMS/EEG revealed a core difference between conscious wakefulness and dreamless sleep, a difference that, theoretically speaking, made perfect sense: no integration, no consciousness. But hold on, maybe neurons are a just little lazier during sleep. Maybe it will be enough to knock a little harder to overcome the blockage, and elicit a widespread and complex echo. In this case, the difference would only be relative and therefore of little interest. To dispel this doubt we decided to repeat the experiment, but this time we turned the stimulator's dial up almost to its maximum intensity, corresponding to an electric field on the cerebral cortex of 160 V/m, virtually a magnetic hummer. The instant we turned on the TMS, an enormous, uniform magnetic wave invaded the student's brain, propagating from the site of stimulation like an oil slick [187]. Every single one of the 60 electrodes recorded the same response, a positive peak in voltage, followed by a negative deflection, a trough as deep as the peak was high. The symphony of wakefulness gave way to a loud thump, and the entire thalamocortical system shuddered like a uniform mass, just like the beating heart or a liquid aggregate of homogeneous elements. We woke our student again and asked the same question. What was going on in your head? The poor fellow opened his eyes, looked at us as if we were aliens from outer space, tormenting him with robot tweezers and probes, shook his head and said "Nothing at all, guys." It was 3 o'clock in the morning and we let him go home.

We repeated the same sequence on a number of subjects and the results were always the same, when we knocked on the awake brain, TMS/EEG invariably revealed a large core of complex causal interactions that disappeared in dreamless sleep. The unconscious brain either reacted with a local slow wave indicating a loss of integration or, when we tried to force a way through using potent stimuli, a global uniform wave

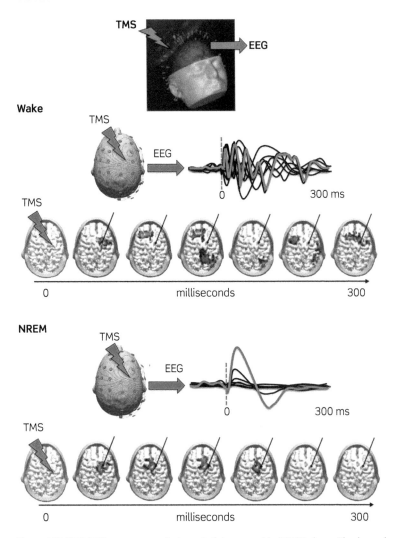

Figure 7.3 TMS/EEG measurements in wakefulness and in NREM sleep. The jagged red arrow indicates the site of stimulation, which is kept constant during the whole measurement by the navigation system (upper panel). The blue circles on the subject's scalp indicate the position of the EEG electrodes. The traces represent the averaged (150 trials) electrical response of the brain recorded by different electrodes (the red trace highlights the activity picked up by the electrode located directly under the stimulator). The seven images depicted below show the spatial–temporal

indicating a loss of information (Figure 7.4). If the shapes and meanings of experience are really woven into the complexity of cause–effect interactions within the brain, it is hardly surprising that the universe disappears, or at least loses its brilliance, when we descend into deep sleep.

Sleep Dreaming

Sleep is the only physiological condition in which a human may cease to exist subjectively, but there are moments in the night when subjective experience returns. Dreams interrupt the void of deep sleep and tend to occur with greater frequency in the later part of the sleep cycle [137]. Oneiric experiences occur very often (but not only) during the REM phase, which is characterized by an acceleration in the EEG trace that shows smaller and more frequent waves, a significant reduction in the peripheral muscle tone (a sort of temporary paralysis), and the appearance of REMs. As we mentioned earlier, REM sleep is also associated with a profound sensory disconnection. Inputs coming from the external environment are not incorporated into the dream experience and are blocked somewhere at the early stages of cortical processing [82, 188], as witnessed by the absence of late event-related responses to sensory stimuli, such as the P3 [189]. Yet subjects are vividly conscious! So, a crucial question is whether it is possible to use TMS/EEG to bypass sensory inputs and motor outputs, and demonstrate the presence of a complex core of causal interactions during

---

dynamics of cortical activation (after source reconstruction) triggered by TMS. During wakefulness, TMS triggers a complex EEG response where many electrodes are involved (high integration) and where each electrode reacts with a different waveform (high differentiation). The corresponding cortical activation is characterized by a long-range, long-lasting pattern of causal interactions where different cortical areas become engaged at different times. During NREM sleep, TMS triggers a large EEG positive–negative wave that is predominant in the electrode placed directly under the stimulator (red trace). The corresponding pattern of cortical activation is a strong, stable current that remains confined to the stimulated cortical module, indicating a break-down of complex causal interactions.

Data from Marcello Massimini, Fabio Ferrarelli, Reto Huber, Steve K. Esser, Harpreet Singh, and Giulio Tononi, Breakdown of cortical effective connectivity during sleep, *Science*, 309(5744), pp. 2228–32, Figure 3. DOI: 10.1126/science.1117256, September 2005.

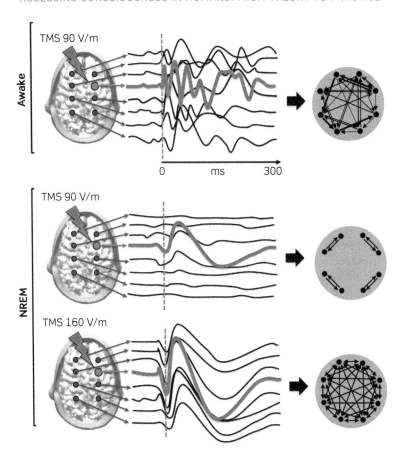

Figure 7.4 During NREM sleep, the brain fails to produce responses that are jointly integrated and differentiated. The jagged red arrow indicates the site of stimulation and the traces show the time-course of TMS-evoked activation recorded at different cortical sites (circles). The red trace highlights the response of the cortical area placed directly under the TMS coil. First row: during wakefulness TMS triggers a pattern of causal interactions that is, at once, integrated and differentiated as it would be expected in the case of the balanced architecture depicted on right. Second row: during NREM sleep, TMS delivered at the same cortical site at the same intensity (90V/m) only elicit a local activation, as it would be expected in the case of the modular system depicted on the right. Third row: increasing stimulation intensity (160V/m) elicits global wave of stereotypical activation that spreads over the cortex, as would be expected in the case of the homogeneous system depicted on the right.

dreaming. With this question in mind, we returned to the sleep laboratory with a strong motivation to catch a dream with our magnetic probe.
It turned out to be a daunting proposition because steady episodes of REM
sleep only come late in the night, at a time when the experimenter is normally exhausted, the contacts between the EEG electrodes and the scalp
are often bad and the TMS coil is overheated. After dozens of frustrating
attempts, one night we positioned once more the TMS/EEG probe and
settled down to wait, with not much hope. After approximately 20 min
the volunteer fell asleep and, once again, we saw the multiform echo of
the conscious brain collapsing into a simple wave. Another 4 h passed as
we waited for the right moment, just like fishermen waiting for the ripple
that indicates the time is right to pull on the line. Then it came! The trace
that recorded electrical activity in the muscles flattened out, while two
major bleeps appeared on the trace recording eye movement. We glanced
at our subject, another university student, who was lying in the reclining
chair, motionless, with his eyes shut. He could neither hear nor speak;
his brain was like a black box, isolated and temporarily inaccessible. We
waited another 10 s and furtively turned on our magnetic dream catcher.
TMS-evoked activity spread and rebounded for a few hundred milliseconds (Figure 7.5), drawing a complex echo on the computer screen [190].
As soon as we were sure we had enough data, we shook the student awake
and asked him the usual question: "What happened? Tell us what was
going on in your head!" This time we got a story, the report was lengthy,
a little confused maybe, but quite articulate; almost 350 words telling of
places, some known to the student others not, a mixed crowd at a party, familiar faces that suddenly transformed into strangers, an ex-girlfriend, and
an intense emotion that we did not investigate further . . . that was enough
for us, we were happy knowing that a universe had returned, entirely generated within the brain—and that we had been able to see its reflection.

In the following year, we spent many nights only to catch another
dozen dreams, but enough to confirm the main result—a conscious report upon awakening can be predicted by the complexity of the brain
echo observed during sleep. Recently, the challenge was taken a step

Data from Marcello Massimini, Fabio Ferrarelli, Steve K. Esser, Brady A. Riedner, Reto Huber,
Michael Murphy, Michael J. Peterson, and Giulio Tononi, Triggering sleep slow waves by
transcranial magnetic stimulation, Proceedings of the National Academy of Sciences of the
United States of America, 104(20), pp. 8496–501, doi: 10.1073/pnas.0702495104, May 2007.

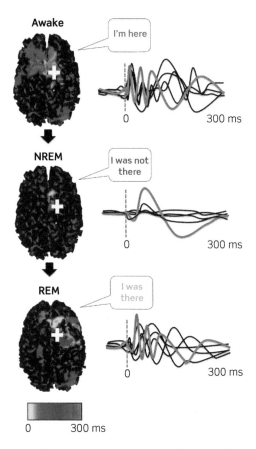

Figure 7.5 Recovery of complex responses during REM sleep. Overnight TMS/EEG measurements are performed in a subject transitioning from wakefulness, to NREM sleep to REM sleep. The brain maps on the left side show the spatial–temporal pattern of cortical activation triggered by TMS in the three states; the colors indicate the latency of activation, from 0 (blue) to 300 ms (red). The traces on the right represent the corresponding EEG scalp responses (the red trace highlights the responses recorded from the sensor located under the stimulator). The presence/absence of consciousness is assessed through a retrospective reports upon awakening (indicated by the balloon "I was there" or "I was not there"). A complex spatial-temporal dynamics recovers upon transitioning from NREM to REM sleep upon awakening from which the subject reports having had a long dream ("I was there").

further by researchers at the University of Wisconsin, who were able to demonstrate a difference in TMS-evoked responses within the same state of NREM sleep, depending on whether subjects reported a dream or not, thus confirming the ability of TMS/EEG to detect a difference in the capacity for experience, everything else being equal [191].

Loss of Consciousness in General Anesthesia

For the past 150 years doctors have been fundamentally agnostic about physical mechanisms of consciousness, but this has in no way hampered the routine use of certain chemical concoctions to annihilate consciousness in patient undergoing surgical procedures. We know empirically that certain molecules extinguish consciousness even if we don't know exactly why. Given the practical success of anesthesiology, the relatively isolated cases of patients who recover consciousness on the operating table seem acceptable. Yet, even these could be avoided if it were possible to find an accurate index to detect recovery of consciousness independently of behavior.

Leaving this question aside for the moment, we can consider general anesthetics from a purely scientific point of view. We have just seen that, in line with theoretical predictions, brain complexity collapses and resurges when consciousness fades and recovers across the sleep–wake cycle, but we do not know yet whether these results can be generalized to other conditions. If a theoretical prediction is general, it must hold for all conditions, including the many ways in which consciousness can be manipulated pharmacologically.

Hence, we designed protocols to obtain TMS/EEG measurements, while subjects were made unconscious by different chemical agents. We started with three commonly used consciousness-annihilators with diverse mechanisms of action—midazolam, propofol, and xenon. There is no need to describe these experiments in detail here, as the main outcome was straightforward; in all such cases, whether the agent was administered by intravenous injection or as a gas through a mask, the

Adapted from, Cortical reactivity and effective connectivity during REM sleep in humans, M. Massimini, F. Ferrarelli, M. J. Murphy, B. Huber, B. A. Riedner, S. Casarotto & G. Tononi, Cognitive Neuroscience, 1(3), pp. 176–83, doi.org/10.1080/17588921003731578. © 2010, Routledge. Reprinted with permission of Taylor & Francis Ltd, http://www.tandfonline.com.

multiform echo observed in wakefulness collapsed into the usual slow wave and subjects reported the usual "I was not there" when prompted upon awakening (Figure 7.6A).

Intriguingly, midazolam, propofol, and xenon, which act by very different pharmacological mechanisms, all resulted in a slow wave that either remained local (pointing to a loss of integration) or propagated like an oil spot (pointing to a loss of information) [192, 193]. If, indeed, consciousness depends on an improbable equilibrium between unity and diversity, it may be easier to understand why, over the centuries, man has found so many compounds that annihilate experience.

Disconnected Consciousness: The Interesting Case of Ketamine

A key goal of anesthesia is to prevent the unpleasant experience of surgery and the most secure way of doing so is to suppress consciousness altogether with deep enough anesthesia. However, an alternate strategy is to enforce a state of disconnection, whereby subjects may retain consciousness, but are completely isolated from the external environment. This condition, called dissociative anesthesia, can be typically achieved through the administration of ketamine [194]. This drug is remarkable in that, at the right dosage, it induces profound disconnection and unresponsiveness, but subjects often report "ketamine dreams" upon emergence from anesthesia [83, 195]. At times, these dreams can turn into really bad trips, thus ketamine is now rarely used, in spite of being a very effective and safe agent. Subjects under ketamine anesthesia are totally unresponsive and, unlike a sleeping subject, cannot be awakened, even with painful stimuli; in fact, they can undergo major invasive interventions. In this respect, ketamine anesthesia takes the sensory disconnection of REM sleep to the extreme, but there is something even more interesting. Behaviorally, there is a striking similarity between this pharmacologically induced condition and the VS/UWS; like brain-injured, unresponsive patents, ketamine-anesthetized subjects show increased muscle tone and lie in their bed open-eyed, with a blank stare, totally unreactive to external stimuli. Practically, if these subjects were to be assessed through a typical bedside testing with the coma recovery scale (CRS), their score would indicate complete unconsciousness. Their spontaneous brain activity, as recorded by the EEG, is also very different from wakefulness; slower rhythms and large amplitude slow waves are prominent, a pattern that is not too different from the one observed during dreamless sleep and other forms of anesthesia [196]. In addition, late brain responses to sensory stimuli, such as the P3, are absent, confirming a strong gating of sensory processing [197–199]. Yet, these subjects are conscious. How do we know that? We know it because, unlike VS/UWS patients, ketamine-anesthetized subjects can tell us where they have been. When the effect of the drug has vanished, subjects can provide retrospective reports that are just like full-fledged dreams, having a highly structured and explicitly narrative, rich emotional components, and being extended in time. These experiences, completely unrelated to the external environment, are sometimes very distressing, at other times pleasant, such as this one, reported by one of our experimental subjects:

[. . .] I had the feeling of falling backwards into space. [. . .] I then found myself in a futuristic spatial vessel-like environment, discussing with two people I know about some abstract theoretical problem I am interested in, and we concluded that there was no solution, and that we disagreed on some fundamental points. The conversation was very intense, but no anger was associated with it. At the end of this brief discussion I came up with the strong conclusion that everything I thought before was wrong, that nothing I believed was true anymore [. . .]. At this stage, the space of my dream became slippery, I fell again with a feeling of shrinking space where everything became oblique, and I could see through the window a very large, white sphere in the intersideral space. [. . .] I continued to fall and arrived in another room, still thinking that I had to find a solution to our theoretical problem using some kind of technology or way of calculation that did not exist yet; I had, at that point, a vision of a futuristic environment with a lot of machines, and some intense discussions with some unknown people about this mathematical problem. Then, reality started to fade and shrink further, the space of my dream flattened and virtually disappeared, and instead there was the apparition of something like a white and bright shape invading progressively the whole space. I would describe this scene as a beautiful end-of-the-world vision, with a real sensation of beauty, very impressive and strange, but no anxiety associated with it [. . .].

All this, and much more, was experienced during our ketamine anesthesia experiments, while the subjects' consciousness was completely inaccessible from the external perspective of an observer. This time around, we had to hold our breath before switching on the stimulator,

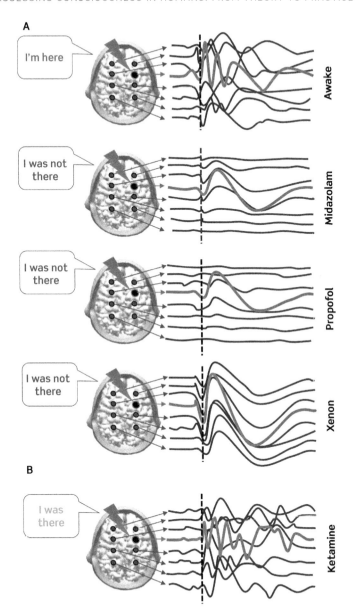

Figure 7.6 Relationships between consciousness and complexity during unresponsiveness induced by anesthesia. (A) The four rows show, from top to

because we knew that this was a critical phase of our endeavor—the final test to validate a measure of consciousness that is independent from sensory processing and motor outputs, or a failure requiring a radical revision of our approach. It turned out that, under the probe of TMS, unresponsiveness induced by ketamine anesthesia was dramatically different from the same behavioral unresponsiveness under midazolam, propofol, and xenon, upon awakening from which subjects reported no experience. Instead of the stereotypical slow wave, under ketamine, the brain returned on the computer screen the multiform echo typical of conscious wakefulness, in spite of a complete disconnection and a sleep-like background EEG [193] (Figure 7.6B).

Finally, we had a way to detect a capacity for consciousness, above and beyond motor behavior, sensory processing, task engagement, and spontaneous brain activity, at least in healthy controls. It was almost time to move our bulky equipment to the bedside of patients emerging from coma, to probe brain islands, and listen to their echo.

Quantifying TMS/EEG Data: The Perturbation Complexity Index

Before moving TMS/EEG to the hospital, however, we had to solve a couple of problems. The first challenge was to transform eyeball descriptions

---

bottom, show the cortical responses evoked by TMS during wakefulness, midazolam, propofol, and xenon anesthesia. The jagged red arrow indicates the site of stimulation and the traces show the time-course of TMS-evoked activation recorded at different cortical sites (circles). In all these cases, subjects lost consciousness as assessed through retrospective reports collected upon awakening ("I was not there") and the complex response of wakefulness collapsed into a stereotypical slow wave. (B) Upon awakening from ketamine anesthesia, subjects reported vivid and intense dreaming; only in this case TMS triggered a complex wakefulness-like response despite complete behavioral unresponsiveness at the time of measurement.

Data from Simone Sarasso, Melanie Boly, Martino Napolitani, Olivia Gosseries, Vanessa Charland-Verville, Silvia Casarotto, Mario Rosanova, Adenauer Girardi Casali, Jean-Francois Brichant, Pierre Boveroux, Steffen Rex, GiulioTononi, Steven Laureys, and Marcello Massimini, Consciousness and complexity during unresponsiveness induced by propofol, xenon, and ketamine, *Current Biology*, 25(23), pp. 3099–105, Figure 2, doi.org/10.1016/j.cub.2015.10.014, November 2015.

and intuitions into quantitative terms, that is, to capture in one number the theoretically relevant aspects of our results. It took some time and thinking until we came up with a method to quantify, albeit coarsely, integrated information starting from TMS/EEG data. Operationally, the procedure involved two fundamental steps. First, extracting the causal effects of TMS in the brain by applying a conservative statistic to TMS-evoked responses in order to obtain a spatiotemporal matrix of significant deterministic cortical activations. Second, compressing this spatiotemporal matrix to calculate its complexity by means of the same algorithms that we use to zip files and images on a computer. Schematically, the procedure involved "zapping" the cortex and "zipping" its responses, thus we called the resulting metrics the perturbational complexity index (PCI) [200]. The underlying idea is that PCI should be low if causal interactions among cortical areas are reduced (loss of integration), because the matrix of activation engaged by TMS is spatially restricted; PCI is also low if many interacting areas react to the perturbation, but they do so in a stereotypical way (loss of differentiation) because in this case the resulting matrix is large, but redundant and can be effectively compressed. In fact, PCI should reach high values only if the initial perturbation is transmitted to a large set of integrated areas that react in a differentiated way, giving rise to a spatiotemporal pattern of deterministic activation that cannot be easily reduced or zipped (Figure 7.7).

It is worth noting that this novel index differs substantially from other metrics that have been previously employed to assess consciousness. Unlike measures of the differentiation of spontaneous activity (entropy, algorithmic complexity), PCI only evaluates the deterministic responses of the cortex to perturbations and is, therefore, largely insensitive to random processes or to patterns that are not generated through causal interactions. Unlike measures of integration that rely on widespread neural synchronization (coherence, phase locking, mutual information), PCI is low when neural activations are spatially extended, but not differentiated. Finally, unlike sensory event-evoked potentials (ERPs) PCI bypasses both sensory inputs and motor outputs, and directly access the core that is relevant for consciousness. In essence, PCI quantifies the amount of irreducible information generated by causal interactions within the thalamocortical system, thus providing an empirically measurable scalar that, albeit crudely, approximates the theoretical measure of Φ as defined in Chapter 5.

(i) Perturb → (ii) Record → (iii) Binarize → (iv) Compress

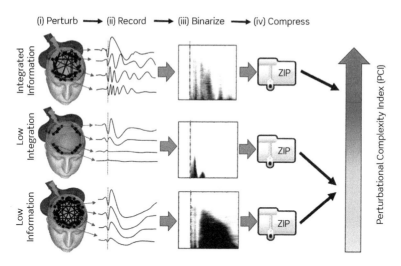

Figure 7.7 PCI simultaneously quantifies integration and differentiation. Operation-ally, calculating PCI involves: (i) perturbing the brain; (ii) recording the cortical response (about 200 trials): (iii) performing statistics to extract a binary matrix describing the spatial-temporal pattern of deterministic, causal interactions; and (iv) compressing (zipping) this matrix. Local (low integration) or stereotypical (low differentiation) responses can be effectively compressed, yielding low PCI values. By contrast, responses that are both integrated and differentiated are less compressible, resulting in high PCI values.

Data from Adenauer G. Casali, Olivia Gosseries, Mario Rosanova, Mélanie Boly, Simone Sarasso, Karina R. Casali, Silvia Casarotto, Marie-Aurélie Bruno, Steven Laureys, Giulio Tononi, and Marcello Massimini, A theoretically based index of consciousness independent of sensory processing and behavior, *Science Translational Medicine*, 5(198), pp. 198ra105, Figure 2, doi: 10.1126/scitranslmed.3006294, August 2013.

Validation and Calibration of PCI

With a theory-based numeric index at hand, we were ready to take the last methodological step. Our goal, and that of much of clinical neuro-physiology, was to find an objective cut-off to detect those patients who retain a capacity for consciousness even in the absence of any evidence based on sensory processing and motor behavior. This task, however, presents an intrinsic challenge, due to a fundamental problem having to do with circular logic. How can we validate an index of conscious-ness in patients who are fully inaccessible and do not provide any reliable evidence about their state of consciousness? Most research studies about brain-based biomarkers of consciousness in coma patients become, sooner or later, stuck in this circular trap [201, 202]. They attempt to validate a marker with an unknown performance on a population, typically including VS/UWS patients, in which the ground truth is also unknown (due to the fallacies of behavioral assessment). One equation with two unknowns, which cannot be solved.

Overcoming this logical short-circuit required a change in perspective and taking a slightly longer way. The change in perspective is that unresponsive patients should not be considered as the population on which the marker has to be validated, but as the individuals to which the marker needs to be applied, possibly to reveal something new about them. The way is longer in that the marker needs to be first validated based on a ground truth, that is, on a control population in which we have strong evidence about the presence or absence of consciousness. With this in mind, we spent time and effort in calibrating the newly developed PCI on a large benchmark population of 150 subjects who could confirm the presence or absence of conscious experience through immediate or delayed reports. This population included:

- healthy subjects of different ages (range 18–80 years) and conscious brain-injured patients who were awake and able to communicate;
- unresponsive subjects who did not report any conscious experience upon awakening from NREM sleep or midazolam, xenon, and propofol anesthesia;
- subjects who were disconnected and unresponsive during REM sleep and ketamine anesthesia, but retrospectively reported having had vivid conscious experiences upon awakening.

Considering subjects' reports as a practical standard for assessing consciousness (no report = unconscious condition; immediate or delayed report = conscious condition), we then performed receiver operating characteristic (ROC) curve analysis. This kind of analysis was developed during World War II, when radar receiver operators were being assessed on their ability to discriminate the presence of incoming enemy aircrafts from harmless sources of signal (e.g., flocks of birds).

Not only did individual radar operators differ in their skills, but changes in the radar receiver gain levels could influence detection; lowering the gain may lead to missing many enemy aircrafts (false negative results), whereas increasing it may lead to many false alarms (false positive results). Thus, the goal of ROC is to assess a test's performance, as well as the optimal threshold that jointly reduced false negative and false positive results.

By applying ROC analysis to assess the ability of PCI to detect consciousness versus unconsciousness, we found an empirical cut-off (PCI = 0.31), which we called PCI*, yielding 100% sensitivity (no false negative results) and 100% specificity (no false positive results) across all the conditions included in the benchmark population (Figure 7.8).

We were particularly satisfied because the PCI radar performed with maximum accuracy even in stress-test conditions, where other empirical measures had not even been assessed before. Indeed, the benchmark population included not only a large group of conscious patients with a heterogeneous set of brain injuries (subcortical and cortical stroke, LIS, and multifocal traumatic injuries), but also the challenging case of conscious subjects disconnected from the environment. Most important, we had an objective threshold. Although we knew that this was not a magic number, nor an absolute boundary between consciousness and unconsciousness, we finally had an operational criterion to guide us in conditions in which no other reference is available. Thus, we pushed our testing further.

Testing PCI at the Boundary of Consciousness: Minimally Conscious Patients

As described in Chapter 3, MCS patients incarnate the boundary of consciousness, the last line of behavioral evidence before the unknown land of the VS/UWS. Even though MCS patients are unable to provide a verbal report about their subjective experience, they show some overt signs of consciousness [203]. The presence of such signs, albeit faint and fluctuating, can be considered as a minimal standard against which the sensitivity of any candidate index of consciousness should be tested. This check is relevant because the reliable detection of MCS patients represents a general challenge for bedside, brain-based indices of

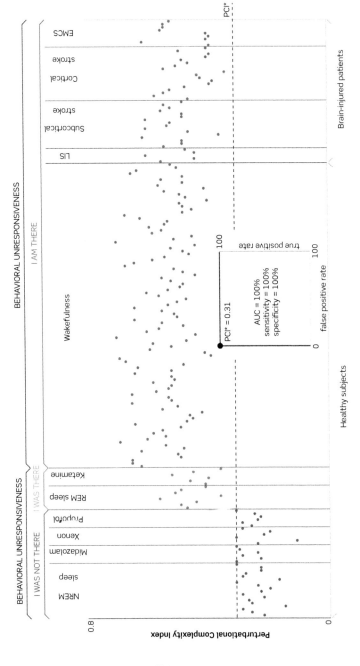

Figure 7.8 Calibration of PCI in the benchmark population. Each circle represents the PCI value computed from the cortical responses to TMS in one subject (for each subject only the session yielding the maximum PCI value is considered). Individuals are grouped by condition and within each condition are sorted by increasing age. During NREM sleep and anesthesia with midazolam, xenon, and propofol, subjects were behaviorally unresponsive and did not provide any report upon awakening ("I was not there"). During dreaming and ketamine anesthesia, subjects were behaviorally unresponsive, but provided delayed subjective reports upon awakening ("I was there"). During wakefulness, both healthy subjects and conscious brain-injured patients could immediately report their subjective experience ("I am here"). The inset shows the result of ROC curve analysis applied to PCI values for computing the optimal cut-off (PCI* = 0.31) that discriminates between unconsciousness (as assessed through the absence of any subjective report) and consciousness (as assessed through the presence of either an immediate or a delayed subjective report). The cut-off PCI* is indicated by the dashed line. Area under the curve (AUC) is 100%; using PCI* as a cut-off, sensitivity and specificity both result in 100%.

EMCS = emergence from minimally conscious state; LIS = locked-in syndrome; REM = rapid eye movement.

Adapted from Stratification of unresponsive patients by an independently validated index of brain complexity, Silvia Casarotto, Angela Comanducci, Mario Rosanova, Simone Sarasso, Matteo Fecchio, Martino Napolitani, Andrea Pigorini, Adenauer G. Casali, Pietro D. Trimarchi, Melanie Boly, Olivia Gosseries, Olivier Bodart, Francesco Curto, Cristina Landi, Maurizio Mariotti, Guya Devalle, Steven Laureys, Giulio Tononi, and Marcello Massimini, *Annals of Neurology*, 80(5) pp. 718–29, Figure 1, doi: 10.1002/ana.24779. © 2016, The Authors. Annals of Neurology published by Wiley Periodicals, Inc., on behalf of American Neurological Association.

consciousness. Besides late ERPs, which can be found only in up to 31% of MCS patients [72], synchrony and entropy-related measures based on spontaneous EEG show the best sensitivity, reaching a maximum of 72% [76]. Having in mind the final goal of detecting consciousness in patients who are totally unresponsive, it is crucial to first make sure that the measurement under consideration is highly sensitive in those patients who actually show some behavioral signs of consciousness. Testing sensitivity in patients who are unable to report is important also for another reason. Although subjective reports about the presence/absence of consciousness in a benchmark population are currently the best available evidence for calibrating a metric of consciousness to be applied to subjects that are unable to report, they are not necessarily always reliable. For example, in certain situations people may be conscious, say during a dream, but subsequently forget their experiences. This intrinsic limitation of introspection may affect ROC analysis and the raise optimal cut-off (PCI*), potentially leading to lower sensitivity in brain injured patients.

As shown in (Figure 7.9A) when tested in MCS patients PCI yielded a sensitivity of 95%; 36 out of 38 patients fell above the threshold of complexity (PCI*) independently derived from the benchmark population. The tangible improvement in sensitivity was a definite confirmation that PCI and its calibration were in a position to reliably detect consciousness, even in the absence of reports [204]. Notably, TMS/EEG revealed complex cortical responses also in MCS patients who were characterized by a severely abnormal spontaneous EEG pattern (Figure 7.9B). Thus, perturbations could detect a core of complexity even below the surface of ongoing EEG waves. Finally, we felt it was time to move beyond the behavioral boundaries of consciousness and use our consciousness radar on the neurological battlefield.

Applying PCI to the Unknown: VS/UWS Patients

In VS/UWS patients, the absence of behavioral signs of consciousness per se cannot be considered as proof of the absence of consciousness. On we saw was quite interesting: by knocking on the brain with TMS we found three distinct modes of brain reactivity, all hiding behind the same clinical label [204].

The first kind of mode was a condition of complete cortical unresponsiveness, whereby TMS failed to elicit any significant neuronal reaction resulting in a flat trace, even when the stimulator was aimed at high intensity and at multiple brain sites (Figure 7.10B, left panel). This complete lack of causal effects necessarily resulted in PCI = 0. In our cohort, this no-response TMS/EEG pattern was only found in post-anoxic patients, that is, in patients who suffered diffuse neuronal death in the cerebral cortex following cardiac arrest. In this case, our radar could only corroborate what was already known, based on structural imaging: the cerebral cortex was largely and irreversibly damaged, and could not return any signal. Accordingly, brain metabolism, as measured by PET, was widely suppressed in the cerebral cortex and in the thalamus, but preserved in the brainstem and cerebellum [205]. Essentially, this no-response TMS/EEG pattern reflected a condition in which the physical substrate of consciousness was structurally destroyed, described by early neurologists as the "apallic syndrome". A note of caution is, however, mandatory. Limitations inherent to the TMS technique prevent mapping of the whole brain, thus small or deep responsive areas may escape the radar.

The second mode was more frequent and much more interesting. In this case, TMS elicited a low-complexity cortical response (PCI < PCI*) that was, in all respects, similar to the one observed during dreamless NREM sleep (Figure 7.10B, central panel). In fact, in most VS/UWS patients stimulating portions of the cortex that were anatomically intact (as assessed by structural imaging) invariably resulted in a large, sleep-like slow wave. This result was intriguing for at least two reasons. First, because it represented a clear-cut dissociation between the mechanisms of arousal and the mechanisms of information integration; indeed, these patients were open-eyed and behaviorally awake, whereas their cortical circuits were unable to engage in complex interactions. Second, because the sleep-like response could be found also in VS/UWS patients who retained large portions of an intact brain (in some cases larger than in MCS patients) raising the question as to why thalamocortical circuits may become stuck in a functional state of low complexity. Why was the physical substrate of consciousness structurally there, but disabled? Was it just functionally unbalanced or blocked? Could we do anything to revert to this pathological sleep-like state and restore complexity? We will come back to these important issues at the end of this chapter.

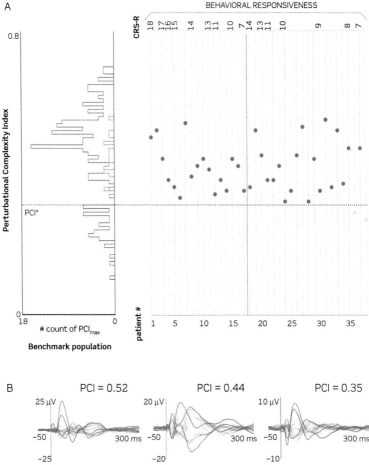

Figure 7.9 Sensitivity of PCI in detecting minimally conscious (MCS) patients. A: The histogram (left) summarizes the distribution of maximum PCI values obtained in the benchmark population in the absence of subjective report (blue) and in the presence of subjective report (delayed, green; immediate, red). The dashed horizontal line

The third mode was most intriguing: in about 20% of VS/UWS patients we found high-complexity responses (PCI > PCI*), that is, the same internal neuronal core that we had learned was associated with the presence of experience, including disconnected dreams (Figure 7.10B, right panel). These instances begged for a thorough reflection. Across hundreds of measurements performed in the benchmark population, PCI was always higher than PCI* when consciousness was present and always below when consciousness was absent, as assessed through subjective report. Moreover, the PCI values found the high-complexity VS/UWS patients were well within the range found in conscious controls. Based on the independent validation of the method, we had to parsimoniously assume that these high-complexity unresponsive patients may have retained a capacity for consciousness that was not expressed in behavior.

---

highlights the optimal cut-off (PCI*) computed from ROC analysis on the benchmark population. The scatter plot (right) shows all the maximum PCI value obtained in individual minimally conscious state (n = 38) patients, sorted by the Coma Recovery Scale-Revised (CRS-R) total score in decreasing order. For each patient, the PCI is represented by a color-filled circle. (B) The first row shows the average TMS-evoked potentials (all channels superimposed, with three illustrative channels highlighted in bold) together with the corresponding PCI values in three representative MCS patients with PCI higher than PCI* (from left to right: Patients 19, 10, and 25). The second row shows 10 s of spontaneous EEG recorded from four bipolar channels (F3-C3, P3-O1, F4-C4, and P4-O2) in the same patients. Despite having all PCI > PCI*, MCS patients displayed patterns of spontaneous EEG activity that were very different: a severely abnormal (left), a moderately abnormal (center), and a mildly abnormal (right) background.

Figure 7.9a: Adapted from Stratification of unresponsive patients by an independently validated index of brain complexity, Silvia Casarotto, Angela Comanducci, Mario Rosanova, Simone Sarasso, Matteo Fecchio, Martino Napolitani, Andrea Pigorini, Adenauer G. Casali, Pietro D. Trimarchi, Melanie Boly, Olivia Gosseries, Olivier Bodart, Francesco Curto, Cristina Landi, Maurizio Mariotti, Guya Devalle, Steven Laureys, Giulio Tononi, and Marcello Massimini, *Annals of Neurology*, 80(5), pp. 718–29, Figure 2, doi: 10.1002/ana.24779. © 2016, The Authors. *Annals of Neurology* published by Wiley Periodicals, Inc. on behalf of American Neurological Association. Figure 7.9b: Adapted from Stratification of unresponsive patients by an independently validated index of brain complexity, Silvia Casarotto, Angela Comanducci, Mario Rosanova, Simone Sarasso, Matteo Fecchio, Martino Napolitani, Andrea Pigorini, Adenauer G. Casali, Pietro D. Trimarchi, Melanie Boly, Olivia Gosseries, Olivier Bodart, Francesco Curto, Cristina Landi, Maurizio Mariotti, Guya Devalle, Steven Laureys, Giulio Tononi, and Marcello Massimini, *Annals of Neurology*, 80(5), pp. 718–29, Figure 3c, doi: 10.1002/ana.24779. © 2016, The Authors. *Annals of Neurology* published by Wiley Periodicals, Inc. on behalf of American Neurological Association.

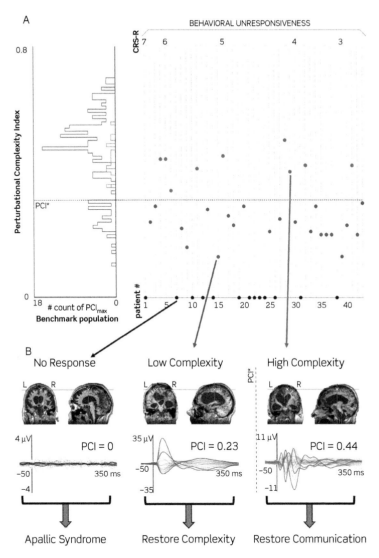

Figure 7.10 PCI-based stratification of unresponsive patients. (A) As in the previous figure, the histogram (left) summarizes the distribution of PCI values obtained in the benchmark population in the absence of subjective report (blue) and in the presence of subjective report (delayed, green; immediate, red) conditions. The dashed horizontal line highlights the optimal cut-off (PCI*) computed from receiver operating characteristic curve analysis on the benchmark population. The scatter

After all, we had just found a similar dissociation between consciousness and behavior in ketamine-anesthetized subjects who lay with eyes open, completely unresponsive at the time of measurement, but had provided a delayed report upon awakening. Unlike these high-complexity anesthetized subjects, high-complexity VS/UWS patients might just be unable to report due to a persistent pathological sensory, motor, or executive disconnection. Perhaps, they all had a capacity for consciousness; whether this was a lucid locked-in state, a dream-like experience, the faint glimpse of falling anesthetized or a full-blown ketamine-like hallucination, we could not know. For some of these patients showing behavioral signs of internal experience was probably just a matter of time, or luck. In fact, it turned out that high-complexity VS/UWS patients had a higher chance (60%) of recovering responsiveness in the months following the measurement compared with ones in the low-complexity mode (20%) and the ones in the no-response mode (0%). Predicting behavioral recovery, however, was not the main point. The point was that we might have detected a capacity for consciousness, an

---

plot (right) shows all the maximum PCI values obtained in individual VS/UWS ($n = 43$) patients, sorted by the CRS-R total score in decreasing order. For each patient, the PCI is represented by a color-filled circle. VS patients could be stratified into three subgroups according to PCI values: high-complexity patients with PCI > PCI* ($n = 9$, red), low-complexity patients with PCI < PCI* ($n = 21$, blue), and no-response patients with PCI = 0 ($n = 13$, black). (B) The structural MRI, the typical average TMS-evoked potential and the corresponding PCI value is reported for a representative subject of each subgroup.

Figure 7.10a: Adapted from Stratification of unresponsive patients by an independently validated index of brain complexity, Silvia Casarotto, Angela Comanducci, Mario Rosanova, Simone Sarasso, Matteo Fecchio, Martino Napolitani, Andrea Pigorini, Adenauer G. Casali, Pietro D. Trimarchi, Melanie Boly, Olivia Gosseries, Olivier Bodart, Francesco Curto, Cristina Landi, Maurizio Mariotti, Guya Devalle, Steven Laureys, Giulio Tononi, and Marcello Massimini, *Annals of Neurology*, 80(5), pp. 718–29, Figure 2, doi: 10.1002/ana.24779. © 2016, The Authors. *Annals of Neurology* published by Wiley Periodicals, Inc. on behalf of American Neurological Association. Figure 7.10b: Adapted from Stratification of unresponsive patients by an independently validated index of brain complexity, Silvia Casarotto, Angela Comanducci, Mario Rosanova, Simone Sarasso, Matteo Fecchio, Martino Napolitani, Andrea Pigorini, Adenauer G. Casali, Pietro D. Trimarchi, Melanie Boly, Olivia Gosseries, Olivier Bodart, Francesco Curto, Cristina Landi, Maurizio Mariotti, Guya Devalle, Steven Laureys, Giulio Tononi, and Marcello Massimini, *Annals of Neurology*, 80(5), pp. 718–29, Figure 4a, doi: 10.1002/ana.24779. © 2016, The Authors. *Annals of Neurology* published by Wiley Periodicals, Inc. on behalf of American Neurological Association.

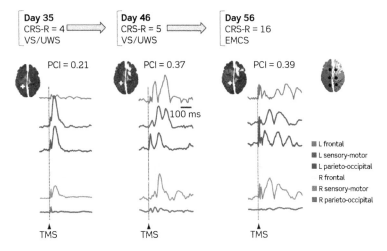

Figure 7.11 Recovery of complexity, before behavioral recovery of consciousness. The figure illustrates the evolution of TMS-evoked responses and PCI in a patient who was followed longitudinally upon awakening from a coma. For each session, the day since injury, CRS-R total scores, and the corresponding clinical diagnosis are indicated. The extent of activation triggered by TMS is plotted on the cortical surface and color-coded, according to their location in six anatomical macro-areas as indicated in the legend; the time-series (colored traces) represent TMS-evoked cortical currents recorded from an array of six sources (black circles on the cortical map in the legend) in each macro-area. The white crosses mark the sites of stimulation in the left parietal cortex.

VS/UWS = unresponsive wakefulness syndrome/vegetative state; EMCS = emergence from the minimally conscious state.

Data from Mario Rosanova, Olivia Gosseries, Silvia Casarotto, Mélanie Boly, Adenauer G. Casali, Marie-Aurélie Bruno, Maurizio Mariotti, Pierre Boveroux, Giulio Tononi, Steven Laureys, and Marcello Massimini, Recovery of cortical effective connectivity and recovery of consciousness in vegetative patients, Brain, 135(4), pp. 1308–20, Figure 2, doi: doi.org/10.1093/brain/awr340, January 2012.

internal core of complexity (or a complex with high Φ), which could not be expressed in behavior. A paradigmatic example is the trajectory of the patient shown in Figure 7.11.

This patient had suffered traumatic brain injury, after which she remained in a coma for 4 weeks. Then, she opened her eyes without giving any behavioral sign of consciousness at the clinical evaluation—the classic VS/UWS. Probing her brain with TMS/EEG at this stage revealed a simple sleep-like response associated with low PCI. A few weeks later the patient seemed to follow for a moment the nurse on duty with her eyes, but this remained an isolated instance that the CRS-R could not objectify; thus, a clinical diagnosis of VS/UWS was confirmed. However, TMS/EEG measurements performed the very same day demonstrated a complex response with PCI > PCI*. This change in the internal state of thalamocortical circuits remained the only evidence that something relevant was happening for another few weeks, until one morning the patient moved her harm towards the nurse and tried to utter some words. Upon request, she raised her hand again and again, nodded to answer questions and made obvious efforts to communicate verbally. Only at this point did the CRS-R jump to scores compatible with a diagnosis of emergence from the MCS. The patient was suddenly able to engage in functional communication. Had she been conscious for weeks? Difficult to say, because she was extremely confused and had serious memory problems. What was clear was that intrinsic brain complexity had been steadily there for weeks, whereas establishing a behavioral channel of communication took much more time and effort on the patient's side.

Sometimes, instead, the burden falls upon the shoulder of the examiner, such as in the case a young boy in his twenties who, after a motorbike accident, had remained behaviorally vegetative for 2 months, upon repeated examinations. During this period, the spontaneous EEG was mixed, but the response to TMS showed the complexity typical of conscious wakefulness in repeated measurements. The case was solved only when his uncle came to visit from north Africa and spoke to him in Arabic, a language the boy had been exposed to only as a young child before moving to Italy at 5 years old—a fact we did not know. The patient smiled, answered questions with gestures, followed his uncle's commands reliably, but kept disregarding instructions in Italian, let alone the boring routine of the CRS-R, which was duly re-administered. The natural conclusion was that he had been conscious throughout; he had just not been interested in showing this to us.

PCI > PCI*: Find a Channel

These two cases we have just described offer an example of how a sensitive objective measure must prompt deeper behavioral investigations. However, other high-complexity patients simply remain in a totally unresponsive state, even after intensive behavioral testing. How do we deal with such cases? Theoretical principles, exhausting benchmark validations, and common sense suggest that we should behave as if these patients are actually conscious, even if they remain unresponsive, even if they have an abnormal EEG, and do not show late ERPs. Since these tests lack sensitivity and can be negative in conscious subjects (for example, during ketamine anesthesia and in MCS patients), we know that their absence in not evidence of the absence of consciousness. It seems more prudent to trust instead the high sensitivity and the high specificity of PCI—an objective measure that has been calibrated against a ground truth—certainly not the perfect truth, but the best available.

In practice, high-complexity VS/UWS patients, in whom the core of internal thalamocortical interactions seem to be in good order, should be selected for intensive interventions aimed at restoring connectedness to the external environment. There are different options here, and cutting-edge approaches are in continuous development. For example, a blockade of motor outputs can be bypassed by active paradigms [66] or brain–machine interfaces based on EEG [206], near-infrared spectroscopy [207], or even intra-cortical recording devices [208]. In these ways, a fully paralyzed patient can learn to modulate his brain activity to answer questions, move computer cursors, or robotic devices. However, applying these techniques is extremely challenging, as it requires extensive training, personalized approaches, and dedicated personnel. Distinguishing among different classes of unresponsive patients through PCI could serve as a principled way to concentrate these resources on those cases in which the physical substrate of consciousness is in working order. Given its sensitivity and specificity, PCI may represent a fundamental screening for a capacity for consciousness, before more complex techniques can be applied to facilitate communication. Beside active paradigms and brain–machine interfaces, more radical interventions are becoming available. An interesting possibility is to increase behavioral output through thalamic stimulations. This invasive approach, which requires implanting electrode in the depth of the brain, boosts the activity of basal ganglia, thereby enhancing the overall excitability of frontal executive and motor circuits [209]. This method has been successfully tested only in MCS patients, but may make a crucial difference in high-complexity VS/UWS patients who are just below the threshold for behavioral manifestations of consciousness. In principle, implantable neuroprosthetic devices may one day help overcome blockages on the input side, also. Preliminary, but encouraging, results have been obtained by direct implants in the occipital cortex to restore rudimentary vision [210] and substantial investments are under way to design implantable devices opening direct, large-band width communication channels between the cortex and external devices [211]. Overall, it seems that the future will be ripe with novel techniques to provide the brain with prosthetic inputs and outputs, and a principled approach to patient selection seems to be a necessary prerequisite. Interventions to restore communication take time, resources, extraordinary efforts, and yet may fail. Once you have confidence, however, that a hidden capacity for consciousness is there, when you have seen its unequivocal, complex echo on the computer screen, it is all worthwhile.

PCI < PCI*: Restore Complexity

As discussed already, unresponsive patients showing high-complexity responses to TMS/EEG call for strenuous efforts to restore inputs and outputs, and thereby communication. What about the large number of low-complexity patients, some of whom may retain large portions of the cortex intact, up to almost one entire hemisphere? Here, the objective to strive for would be to attempt to restore sufficient levels of complexity, under the assumption that the residual neural structure is still capable of doing so. In these brain-injured subjects, the brain's electrical reaction to the TMS perturbation is, at least superficially, indistinguishable from the one observed during dreamless NREM sleep—the usual stereotypical slow wave. Thus, understanding how complexity collapses in the brain of naturally sleeping subjects is the necessary first step for investigating possible ways of helping brain-injured patients.

Why does a majestic piece of architecture, like the waking thalamo-cortical system, collapse into an amorphous and fragmented mass upon falling asleep? How can the brain's capacity for information integration drop in the space of a few minutes, structural connections and average activity levels being roughly the same? Interestingly, a small change in internal neuronal dynamics may make the fatal difference. As already mentioned in Chapter 3, it is well known that, at the level of cortical neurons, the key difference between wakefulness and NREM sleep is an increase in the opening of potassium channels [135]. The resulting currents tend to strongly hyperpolarize neuronal membranes because potassium ions, which carry a positive charge, exit the cells in large amounts. Importantly, these potassium currents are activity-dependent, in that they become stronger with the amount of prior activation. The end result is that, during sleep, cortical neurons develop the tendency to fall into a short period of deep hyperpolarization and complete silence, lasting a few hundred milliseconds, after an initial activation. This simple dynamic is called bistability, because neurons naturally tend to alternate between two extreme states: an active period—otherwise called up-state—and a silent period—otherwise called down-state. This alternation is known to underlie the occurrence of spontaneous slow waves during NREM sleep, but the intriguing possibility is that neuronal bistability may be the key reason why the brain's capacity for integrated information collapses [212].

In a recent experiment we have moved one step closer to neurons to test this hypothesis. We did so by replicating the logic of TMS/EEG measurements, this time inside the cranium. The experiments involved single-pulse intracortical electrical stimulation (SPES in lieu of TMS) and local field potential (LFP) recordings (in lieu of EEG) in humans undergoing presurgical evaluation for the removal of an epileptic focus. As in the case of TMS/EEG experiments, cortical stimulations and recordings were performed both during wakefulness and NREM sleep [213]. The difference was that LFP recordings, unlike EEG traces, could provide more precise information about the behavior of neurons.

As hoped, intracranial measurements provided valuable insights. First, they confirmed TMS/EEG results by showing that during wakefulness electrical stimulation triggers a chain of recurrent deterministic activations in distant cortical targets, whereas during NREM the same input induces a low-complexity slow wave. Second, they revealed the neuronal underpinning of this positive–negative slow wave: in response to SPES, cortical neurons engage in a brief response, then quickly plunge into a silent down-state. This was clear evidence pointing to a bistable behavior, but there was something even more interesting—after the down-state, neuronal activity resumed stochastically, in a way that was totally unrelated to the initial input, whereas during wakefulness large-scale causal effects were prolonged for up to 500 ms. Overall, the picture was clear and consistent: during sleep, due to their tendency to fall into a down-state after an initial activation, cortical neurons become unable to engage in reciprocal complex pattern of causal interactions; upon receiving an input, they tend to respond briefly, then hush, and forget (Figure 7.12). The shift to this bistable behavior is a small step for individual neurons but makes a giant difference under the lens of Φ: first, the occurrence of a stereotypical down-state reduces information capacity (all neurons react in the same way), then the causal chain is interrupted (all neurons resume activity stochastically) leading to a loss of integration. Basically, when the system becomes bistable any input or local activation within the brain can only induce a feed-forward sweep of activation that quickly dissipates into nothing.

Perhaps this is how the marvelous complexity of the entire thalamocortical system can melt upon falling asleep, anatomical structure and average activity levels being fundamentally unchanged! It is a sobering thought; all it takes may be a simple change in potassium conductance, and what took millions of years of natural selection, 9 months of gestation, and a lifetime of experience to create, is suddenly gone.

Of course, in physiological conditions, complexity can be easily restored: a few seconds before we wake up, the neurons of brainstem activating systems increase their firing rates watering the whole thalamocortical system with a cocktail of neurotransmitters, such as acetylcholine, noradrenaline, glutamate, and histamine, that all converge on one single mechanism—closing potassium channels on neuronal membranes [214]. In this way, bistability is gone and complexity recovers in the brain. Sometimes, such as during REM sleep, a whiff of acetylcholine is enough to do the magic, and the universe appears in a dream. This is what seems to happen when consciousness fades and returns across the physiological wake–sleep cycle.

In some pathological cases, instead, switching on the brainstem will not do, even though large portions of the thalamocortical system are spared by the lesion. Why in many VS/UWS patients, cortical areas that are anatomically intact, active, and reactive remain stuck in a low-complexity state? The answer may be that some lesions may precipitate whatever is left of the cortex in a state of pathological sleep-like bistability. Interestingly, this may happen in many different ways, thus pointing to a final common pathway to loss of consciousness. For example, injuries in the depth of the brain may simply interrupt the fibers that convey the activating cocktail from the brainstem to the thalamus and cortex. In such extreme cases, the physical substrate of consciousness may be fully intact, but totally disabled and stuck in a pathological bistable state due to

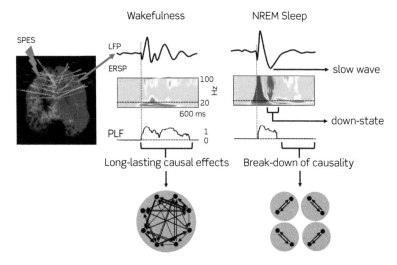

Figure 7.12 Neuronal bistability breaks off causality and information integration during NREM sleep. The figure illustrates the results of experiments involving intracortical single pulse electrical stimulation (SPES) and local field potential (LFP) recordings in humans during wakefulness and NREM sleep. For each condition (wakefulness, NREM sleep), the average SPES-evoked LFP response is shown, together with the corresponding event-related spectral perturbation (ERSP) and the time course of the phase-locking factor (PLF). During wakefulness, electrical stimulation triggers a complex LFP response associated with a long-lasting chain of deterministic effects, as reflected by sustained (~500 ms) PLF in distant cortical targets. During NREM the same input induces a slow wave associated with a cortical down-state (suppression of power >20 Hz in the ERSP, reflecting a period of neuronal silence). After the down-state, cortical activity resumes to wakefulness-like levels, but the phase-locking (PLF) to the stimulus is lost, indicative of a break in the cause-effect chain. Thus, cortical circuits, upon receiving an input, tend to respond briefly, then hush and forget. Overall, these findings suggest that bistability—the tendency of cortical neurons to fall into a down-state after an initial activation—plays a key role in disrupting the cause–effect repertoire of the brain and thus its capacity for integrating information.

Data from Andrea Pigorini, Simone Sarasso, Paola Proserpio, Caroline Szymanski, Gabriele Arnulfo, Silvia Casarotto, Matteo Fecchio, Mario Rosanova, Maurizio Mariotti, Giorgio Lo Russo, J. Matias Palva, Lino Nobili, and Marcello Massimini, Bistability breaks-off deterministic responses to intracortical stimulation during non-REM sleep, *NeuroImage*, 112, pp. 105–13, doi. org/10.1016/j.neuroimage.2015.02.056, May 2015.

lack of critical levels of activating neuromodulation [215]. In other cases, lesions may alter the excitation/inhibition balance in the rest of the cortex in favor of inhibition [216]. This loss of balance is known to occur locally after a stroke, but may involve the whole remaining cortex after a severe, multifocal injury. Crucially, shifting the equilibrium toward excessive inhibition also results in a bistable, low-complexity condition; after all, this is what most anesthetics, such as midazolam and propofol, do (xenon instead, does so by increasing potassium currents). Another experimental way to induce full-blown bistable dynamics is severing a critical amount of white matter fibers below the cortical surface. Intracellular recordings in animal models have shown that, following a surgical white matter undercut (cortical slab), pyramidal neurons develop a stronger tendency to fire briefly and then enter into a silent down-state [217]. In humans, variable degrees of white matter disconnection, known as diffuse axonal injury, often occurs following the accelerations/decelerations associated with traumatic events. Once engendered, bistable dynamics in cortical neurons would result in a global state of functional disconnection and low-complexity, which goes well beyond the share of structural disconnection directly caused by the actual white matter lesion.

To the extent that pathological sleep-like bistability represents a common functional endpoint, disrupting large-scale interaction across structurally intact portions of the cortex, its reduction may be relevant for recovery. The course of events illustrated in Figure 7.13 is compatible with this hypothesis. This figure illustrates the results of longitudinal TMS/EEG measurements performed in one patient evolving from VS/UWS to recovery of consciousness. In this patient, the process of behavioral recovery was associated with a progressive decrease of bistability and by a concurrent recovery of causality and complexity, brain structure being equal [218].

Can we optimize neuromodulation or pharmacological therapeutic strategies to push neurons beyond the threshold for bistable dynamics, thus recovering complexity? In the years to come, it will be crucial to further elucidate the relationships between neuronal bistability, overall network complexity and consciousness through extensive experiments across species and models, including in vitro preparations and large-scale detailed computer simulations.[1] As a preliminary proof of principle, a

---

1 This thorough exploration is one of the several challenges taken up by the Human Brain Project, a 10-year research project launched in 2013 by the European Commission.

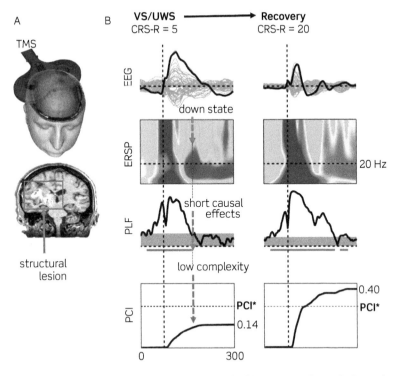

Figure 7.13 Reduction of bistability is associated with recovery of complexity and consciousness in VS/UWS patients. The figures show the results of two subsequent (30 days apart) TMS/EEG measurements in one patient who recovered consciousness from the VS/UWS. (A) the position of the TMS coil is shown (top) together with a coronal section of the MR image showing the location and the extent of the structural lesion: a right frontotemporo-parietal hemorrhage with ischemic sequelae and thalamic hematoma. (B) The evolution of the evoked response (EEG), bi-stability (ERSP), causality (LFP), and complexity (PCI) is shown during the spontaneous process of recovery. Similarly to what shown in Figure 7.12 during sleep, the VS/UWS condition is characterized by an EEG slow wave associated with a cortical down-state (suppression of power >20 Hz in the ERSP), which curtails the causal effects of the initial activation (short-lasting PLF). Crucially, the timing of the down-state (red, dashed arrow) corresponds to the time at which complex neuronal interactions stop building up (as indicated by the plateau of the PCI time course). Upon recovery of consciousness, the down-state disappears, causal interactions are uninterrupted and PCI can grow above the threshold (PCI*) identified in the benchmark population.

recent study employing electrical perturbations and recordings in iso-lated cortical slices (an extreme case of cortical island) showed that com-plex causal interactions, as assessed by an adapted version of PCI, can be manipulated restored by pharmacological manipulations that reduce neuronal bistability [219].

The stakes are high because while bistability can disable the entire thalamocortical system, it can be reversed, at least in principle. This may work in only a selected minority of patients, but it is a possibility that it is worth considering. In fact, in some cases, cortical circuits may just need a little kick. After all, the biological brain and its neurons are plenty of non-linear dynamics, such as voltage-gated channels, spiking thresholds, dendritic amplification, and the like. You close just one more potassium channel, reduce inhibition below a critical level or depolarize a notch the membrane, and the complexity of the whole system may change. This non-linearity may be the reason why complexity, which in theory can go across many subtle gradations, in practice is either high or low: mostly, we all fall asleep, become anesthetized and wake up. Perhaps it is also the reason why some patients spontaneously flip from a low-complexity condition to a conscious high-complexity state with no apparent reason. Whether we will be able to understand and promote this process is an open question, one that we shall try address, having solid principles and the right measuring tools at hand.

This was a rather heavy chapter in which we overloaded the reader with an electrophysiological tour-de-force. Clearly, the story is far for been closed: recording brain responses to TMS in patients still requires a complex equipment, substantial time and man-power. A simplifica-tion of the technique and a standardization of the procedures is war-ranted before PCI can walk out of the research lab towards the routine clinical environment. Even then, the measurement would remain quite crude, a blurred echo from a distant planet. Hopefully, better tech-niques will become available to stimulate and record from the brain on a finer spatial scale, leading to a better approximation of Φ. Although

Data from Mario Rosanova, Matteo Fecchio, Silvia Casarotto, Simone Sarasso, Adenauer G Casali, Andrea Pigorini, Angela Comanducci, Francesca Seregni, Guya Devalle, Olivier Bodart, Melanie Boly, Olivia Gosseries, Steven Laureys, and Marcello Massimini Sleep-like bistability, loss of causality and complexity in the brain of Unresponsive Wakefulness Syndrome patients. *bioRxiv* doi: http:// dx.doi.org/ 10.1101/ 242644, January 2018.

here we have focused on a perturbational approach that was directly driven by IIT's postulates, other methods are being developed that gauge functional differentiation and functional integration in the brain. For example, a recent study has demonstrated that the repertoire (differentiation) of fMRI functional connectivity (integration) configurations is greater during wakefulness than during propofol anesthesia in monkeys [220]. Another work in monkeys showed that electrocortical dynamics become more stable upon loss of consciousness, regardless of anesthetic-specific effects on activity [221]. Likewise, network analysis and computational modeling applied to human fMRI data have suggested that large-scale dynamics and connectivity during loss of consciousness depart from a critical state toward more stable fluctuations [222]. Hopefully novel algorithms [223–227] and modeling approaches [165, 228] based on the analysis of spontaneous brain activity may afford an accuracy similar as the one of PCI, albeit with a simpler set-up. For now, we can conclude that translating basic theoretical principles into empirical measurements offered mechanistic insight and a clear practical advantage. Extensive testing showing high sensitivity and high specificity against a ground truth validate theoretical predictions and indicates that we may be one step closer to the physical substrate of consciousness, allowing for better inference in unknown conditions. A radar that works better than another against a clear blue sky, can also be trusted more when it is pointed at the clouds.

CHAPTER 8

INFERRING CONSCIOUSNESS OUT THERE

As is often the case in science, a theory is first tested and validated in situations that are close to ideal, and then extrapolated to more remote cases. Thus, whether consciousness varies with a system's capacity for integrated information would first be validated on my own consciousness: for example, does Φ, or a surrogate measure, systematically collapse when I undergo general anesthesia or when I fall into a dreamless sleep, and return to high values when we dream or hallucinate during ketamine? Then, one can test other healthy subjects who are able to report and finally extrapolate to more difficult cases, such as to unresponsive patients with islands of functioning brain tissue, as we have done in Chapter 7. In this chapter, we would like to apply the same principle to explore its implications for the physical world outside the human skull. In essence, we shall ask whether and where in nature there are physical mechanisms that are well suited to account for experience, as we know it. We understand this is a reckless proposition, since available empirical measures are obviously not up to the task, but we believe it is a good exercise. Often, the most we can do is to draw our best inferences about unknown instances based on a principle that works well in many known instances, and that it is much better than to make arbitrary claims or to draw no inference whatsoever.

Criteria and Boundaries

In 1970, the biologist Jacques Monod wrote a lucid and visionary essay "Chance and necessity: an essay on the natural philosophy of modern biology," which became a classic of scientific literature. Monod opened with a provocative question, "If we were to land on Mars (or if Martians were to land on Earth), with the objective of searching for traces of some intelligent life form, what should we (they) look for?" His suggestion was that, for a start, the scientists of the space agency who had been entrusted with the mission should search the surface of the planet for some form of organized activity, for the production of artifacts (the product of an activity, of an art form). The first lines of the essay read:

> The difference between artificial and natural objects seems immediately and unambiguously apparent to all of us. A rock, a mountain, a river, or a cloud—these are natural objects; a knife, a handkerchief, a car—so many artificial objects, artifacts. Analyze these judgements, however, and it will be seen that they are neither immediate nor strictly objective.

In the pages that follow, Monod showed just how challenging it is to write a program for a computer that would allow it to distinguish, based on purely objective criteria, which objects are natural in origin and which are artifacts. He points out that the machine should be able to recognize objects of a regular shape automatically, because regularity (right angles, straight lines, perfect symmetry, etc.) is rarely seen in objects carved by natural forces. Then the program should look for repetition, because if the researcher (whether human or alien) were to find symmetrical objects in great numbers (as, for example, Neolithic arrow heads) this would indicate the passage of an organized form of life, with a systematic project, capacity for abstraction, objectives, and goals. Perfect, we couldn't agree more. Then he brings an alien team to Earth to search for an organized life form. They encounter a swarm of bees. Bees are incredibly sophisticated, perfectly symmetrical, and are found in vast numbers; in addition, at least to the human (and probably also to the alien) eye, they seem to be perfect replicas one of the other. At this point their computer tells the aliens that they are in the presence of a highly organized industrial civilization that makes their own attempts back home look like child's play, which produces miniature artifacts of extraordinary complexity in vast numbers. So, are bees artificial or natural? Monod has used this expedient of the tale of the alien expedition to point out a rather startling fact—distinguishing the natural from the artificial, the animated from the unanimated is not as easy as we might think. If a computer has to make this distinction, it has to be programed to consider not only the symmetry and the replication of the objects, but also their origin. While artificial objects (such as arrow heads and digital cameras) are produced by external forces, natural objects like bees and flowers are self-producing, through a process that Monod defined as "autonomous morphogenesis." Once the program has been upgraded to include this variable in its calculations, the problem seems to be taken care of and the alien mission proceeds on its way, but then it comes across a colony of quartz crystals, perfectly symmetrical, faithfully replicated, which multiply by autonomous morphogenesis. The alien team at this point are really perplexed. What is the criterion that distinguishes the crystal from a living being? According to Monod, it is a question of quantity, not quality. The difference lies in the quantity of information that organizes the growth of the object, not the quality. Only minimal information is required to repeat the elementary cell of the crystal, a bit more to code for the structure of a virus and a myriad to form a biological cell. The essay continues with a fascinating journey through the molecular structure of the DNA to alight at the organization of human society, but here we will leave Monod and the problem of characterizing living forms. The point is simply that, even basic distinctions that we take for granted, such as that between living and not living, can be extremely difficult to pin down on the basis of objective criteria.

Plotting a Chart

Now, keeping in mind that the divide between the inanimate and the animate is not as clear as it may seem at a first glance, let us move on to the problem of the presence of consciousness outside the human head. In this case, we ourselves are the visiting aliens, born and bred on a planet of which we know very little. The issue is now in the following terms— How do we recognize the presence of "someone who feels something" in a world populated by an incredible variety of beings that are not in a position to communicate their experiences to us?

Let's try to transform this question into chart form. We will put all biological and non-biological objects that populate the planet on the x-axis. We could put them in random order, but just for the sake of narration we will sort them roughly into their reverse phylogenetic order. First come humans, then apes and other terrestrial mammals, then marine mammals, birds, reptiles, amphibians, invertebrates, mushrooms, plants, bacteria, and so on. We don't want to leave anything out, so we will add inanimate objects, such as crystals, stones; human artifacts, such as GPS navigators, smartphones, and computers. Primary consciousness goes onto the y-axis. What do we mean by primary consciousness? The sensation we experience when watching the landscape passing by through the window of the train, when we are completely absorbed by the plot of a film, or remain captivated by the sound of the waves rippling onto the shore and the play of light on their crests; that is, anything that doesn't require a special effort of reflection, attention, memory, imagination, or choice [229]. Perhaps only those who have practiced meditation as a rigid discipline for years can assess properly whether it is possible for a human being to shake of the weight of all reflections, self-awareness, and effortful thinking [230], but what we can all say with a satisfactory degree of certainty is that that weight may be much reduced when experiencing pure dark, a color, a flower, appreciating the purity of a sound, a perfume or enduring pain.

Once we have roughly defined the variables of the axes, we can entertain a few interesting questions. Let's start by asking how the capacity to feel pain (say, a pinprick) is distributed along our x-axis. Of course, we could have considered the experience of pleasure, or the experience of light or dark. We chose pain as it is more effective in stressing the sense of ethical urgency related to the problem of assessing the capacity for consciousness in non-human beings. What would this chart look like? Will it have a peak around humans and then fall precipitously to zero in all the other categories? Or will it be a straight horizontal line, a constant across all categories? A trend that plunges suddenly at the divide between the animate and the inanimate worlds? A curve with a more gradual profile? Or maybe none of these, but a bizarre landscape with multiple valleys and peaks? Well, at present, we just don't know. What we can say is that how we answer these questions should condition the way we interact with the other inhabitants and objects that populate our planet.

In 1974, the American philosopher Thomas Nagel asked the question "What is it like to be a bat?" [231] with the aim of throwing light on the issue of privacy and inviolability of subjective experience. It has become a classic in the philosophy of mind. We certainly do not know what it feels like to explore the intricate depths of a wood winging through branches with only sonar to guide us, but the real problem is that we are not even sure about whether it feels anything at all to be a bat. In fact, we do not have a clear and shared idea of how the capacity for consciousness is distributed throughout the objects in the world, including animals. The basic issue is, of course, that they don't speak, or more precisely, that they do not use a language to which we are privy. Since we are accustomed to attribute consciousness to beings that speak and communicate about their internal states, we are immediately at a disadvantage when faced with the absence of a language that we can decode. Thus, opinions vary in the extreme depending on whom one asks, and this uncertainty has remained unchanged over the centuries. See, for example, the radical divergence between the ideas expressed by two great French philosophers, Descartes and Montaigne.

Descartes drew a sharp line between humans and the rest of the natural world. According to him, verbal and non-verbal language, and logical reasoning are the distinguishing factors that separate man from all the other species. Relying on the principle of parsimony (the famous Occam's razor), the French philosopher maintained that the behavior of all non-human animals can be explained without calling consciousness into play. According to Descartes, the actions of animals, however surprising and complex they may seem, are to be interpreted in purely mechanical terms. Just like the machines produced by mankind, animals are machines produced by Nature. In his Discourse on Method [232], Descartes concluded that animals are just mechanisms that are incapable of any feeling whatsoever:

> [. . .] it is Nature which acts in them, according to the disposition of their organs. Similarly, people recognize that a clock, which is composed only of wheels and springs, can count the hours and measure time more accurately than we can with all our practical wisdom.

Descartes was the first to perfect the system of orthogonal axes (x, y), which still carries his name today. Then, how would he have plotted the chart of primary consciousness (y-axis) versus the objects of the world (x-axis)? Presumably, as a huge peak corresponding to humans that falls back to zero everywhere else. Very neat and tidy, but how would Descartes have classified those millions of patients who lie motionless in the neurological wards and rehabilitation centers, human beings endowed with consciousness, but who have lost the power of speech and, sometimes, of reason? Where would he have positioned those who have not yet acquired the capacity to use speech to communicate? On which side of the barrier would he have placed a child who has not yet learned how to communicate his/her thoughts? Does this same child, after acquiring the faculty of language, suddenly gain an intrinsic perspective, her world becoming populated with colors, forms, sounds, joys, and sorrows? These are just a few of the problems that arise if, like Descartes, we decide to draw a sharp line between the conscious and the unconscious world based on the ability to think and communicate.

Just a few years earlier and not far away, Michel de Montaigne formulated a position diametrically opposed to Descartes [233]. A strong advocate of doubt and cultural relativism, Montaigne loathed clear-cut distinctions and directly opposing positions, by far preferring skepticism. When he dealt with the question of the distribution of consciousness in nature, he characteristically left all the possibilities open:

> [...] when I am playing with my cat, how do I know that she is not passing time with me rather than I with her? [...] Why do we assume it is a defect in the animals and not in us that we cannot communicate with them? We do not understand them any more than they understand us. They may think of us as brute beasts for the same reasons as we think of them to be so [...].

Montaigne could be just as radical as Descartes, however, albeit in a different direction:

> [...] there is a greater difference between a man and another man than between an animal and a man.

Montaigne, with his ecumenical approach that embraced the concept of consciousness for all living organisms enjoys a certain following today. Take Peter Singer, for example, a contemporary Australian philosopher and animal activist pioneer, who draws the line between shrimps and oysters (and mussels), for the delight of the palates of the better-off, and claims, like Montaigne, that some animals may have a greater capacity for consciousness than some humans [234]. Other contemporary thinkers have gone a step further, sustaining the view that consciousness as we experience it is a property that is shared by single cells.

The objective of this brief historical digression, which is obviously incomplete, is just to give an idea of the range of possible positions regarding how consciousness is distributed in nature. It is certainly worthy of note that the range is just as wide today as it was in the times of Montaigne and Descartes. If you ask for an informal view, most people will say that for them inanimate objects are not conscious, and only some living beings are endowed with consciousness. Very few people think that bacteria, mushrooms or plants have any form of consciousness, and worms and leaches don't fare much better. The debate becomes more heated when the subject matter moves up the scale to fish, amphibians, and reptiles, and can become ferocious when birds and mammals are discussed. How many owners of cats or horses would question the capacity of these animals to perceive pain? How many dog owners would question the capacity of their pets to feel not only pain, but happiness and empathy? On the other hand, there are those who maintain that there is no evidence of subjective experience in the animal kingdom, with the exception of man and (maybe) the great primates. To summarize, if we were to conduct a survey among representatives of the human race from different cultures, social extraction, and religion, and asked them to draw the line on our chart of the distribution of primary consciousness, we would end up with many different versions, often radically different. Like Monod's explorers, we need to converge on some objective criteria. Which ones? The current approach to the problem typically relies on two observable properties—either the complexity of behavior or the size of the brain [235]. It is worth trying to draw a chart based on these criteria.

Behaviors

It is perfectly reasonable to hypothesize a connection between the capacity for complex behavior and the capacity for consciousness. The simple fact that our capacity to interact significantly with the world around us decreases when the level of consciousness diminishes during sleep or when we are under the effect of an anesthetic, seem to support this view [236]. Indeed, up to a point the observation of behavior may certainly provide a rough indicator of the presence of consciousness, not only in humans, but also within the animal kingdom [237]. It is a fact that the more carefully we observe animals, the greater the variety and flexibility of their behavior appear, and this is not only true for primates, but also for animals that are phylogenetically far removed from the human species, such as crows, parrots, octopuses, and bees. There is little doubt that these animals, aliens who live in bodies and eco-systems so different from ours, constitute the most interesting challenge of all; so, we will start by examining their behavior patterns, moving from left to right on the x-axis until we reach the great divide between animate and inanimate entities.

Let's start with dolphins. There is a wealth of scientific and popular literature on the behavior of these animals. Whoever has visited a dolphin house will have been able to form an opinion on the capacity of these marine mammals to understand complex verbal instructions, to imitate, learn elaborate motor sequences and work out creative solutions. What is more surprising and has greatly impressed scientists working with dolphins is the complexity of their social interactions when they are in their natural habitat [238]. These mammals seem to be particularly attentive to social dynamics; indeed, they seem to be almost obsessed with them. They live at an exhausting rhythm, weaving relationships, creating alliances, shifting alliances, and betraying their allies. Dolphins see very little with their eyes, they use echo-location instead, in much the same way as bats do. Not only do they monitor the area in which they are swimming, they also eavesdrop the return of the impulses emitted by other dolphins, to get an idea of what they are seeing. Marine biologists are coming to the conclusion that, behind what appears to us to be a playful and happy-go-lucky existence, dolphins are actually involved in a social whirl, which is perhaps more intricate and, at times, paranoid than many human associations. It seems that dolphins, like humans and the great apes, can recognize themselves in a mirror, which is a behavior that for many psychologists suggests the presence of self-consciousness. That said, it is extremely difficult to interpret the behavior in front of a mirror of a dolphin, a being without hands or facial mimics, much more difficult than, say, interpreting that of a monkey. This is one of the reasons why the question of self-awareness in dolphins is still a subject of debate [239]. On the other hand, the most articulate behavior is not necessarily the most indicative: sometimes dolphins blow bubbles, then they move off a little distance and turn to watch them dancing up through the water. Why do they do this? A well-deserved break from an exhausting social life? A fresh breath of primary consciousness? Unfortunately, dolphins cannot talk to us and so we just don't know.

There are other animals that do talk to us. Parrots, for example. Take the case of Alex, an African Grey who was trained over a period of approximately 30 years by the American researcher Irene Pepperberg [240]. Towards the end of his life, Alex had acquired a vocabulary of 150 words (similar to the vocabulary of a 2-year old human), he could count up to six, distinguish seven colors, and six geometric forms, and had even a grasp of some general concepts, such as "bigger," "smaller," "same," "different," "above," "below," and "zero." He was able to categorize objects, like keys, independently of their color, material, or form, and when he was tired, he would say, "wanna go back," which certainly gave the lie to the common saying, "learn like a parrot." Alex died unexpectedly in 2007 and his successors have not revealed the same level of ability. Now, what would Descartes have said if he had been able to meet Alex? Other birds don't speak, but show behavior that we consider to be typically human, such as the ability to make and use utensils. The crows of New Caledonia, for example, have been known to bend a hair pin to make a hook that they use to extract food from a cylindrical container [241], a type of activity that reveals a noteworthy capacity for discrimination and planning. Another interesting research study in 1995 assessed the ability of certain pigeons to recognize and distinguish the works of Picasso and Monet [242]. After training they were able to distinguish paintings by these artists, even if they had never seen the paintings before. Quite amazing!

Going further right on our scale, we come to the octopus, a marine mollusc with eight limbs and three hearts that would not look out of place in a far-fetched science fiction film. Is it really worthwhile investigating the consciousness of this cephalopod that lives a solitary existence among the rocks on the sea bed? Consider that *Octopus vulgaris* has a range of extraordinarily flexible behaviors, supported by a significant working memory and highly developed discrimination abilities [243]. It is able to distinguish artifacts of different weights, forms, and dimensions, it uses objects such as stones and the shell of the coconut to procure food, to hide, to play, and is able to learn the best strategy (among many) to find a way out of a maze. Although octopuses are not social beings, they have an extraordinary capacity to learn from their fellows: an octopus that observes its neighbor in a nearby in aquarium opening a jar to extract food, can immediately imitate the same movements as soon as it is given a similar jar [244]. In addition, they seem to be mischievous and sneaky—they can systematically squirt their ink on selected people who they do not like and do overnight raids of neighboring tanks for food [245]. Given these abilities, and much more besides, entire books and essays have been dedicated to the wondrous nature of octopuses [245–247]. Even more, cephalopods have been the subject of UK and EU protective legislation "as there is scientific evidence of their ability to experience pain, suffering distress and lasting harm."

Moving further right on our axis we come across a swarm of bees, like the one encountered by Monod's alien explorers. The social behavior of these insects (division of labor, construction, and maintenance of the beehive, castes, and task differentiation depending on age) is notoriously complex. Not unlike dolphins, bees live in highly stratified, yet flexible social organizations with group decision-making skills that rival academic or corporate committees in efficiency. Although many of the aspects of the bees' social behavior are somewhat rigid as they are genetically predetermined, bumble bees can show a surprising degree of cognitive flexibility in, for example, manipulating objects [248]. However, bees have other well-known remarkable abilities, such as that of communicating distances and coordinates of food sources to other bees with extreme precision. This communication is done by a figure 8 "waggle dance," during which the bee performs waggling movements [249]. Flowers located in line with the sun are indicated by a waggling run in an upward direction, and any angle to the right or the left of the sun is coded with a corresponding angle to the right or left of the upward direction. The distance between the hive and the recruitment target is encoded in the duration of the waggle runs. The further away is the food source, the longer the waggle, with an increase coefficient of approximately 75 ms for every 100 m. Apparently more expert bees, the ones who have been in the hive longest, are even capable of adjusting the angulation of their waggle dance to take into consideration the movement of the sun, so that the additional help is able to find the food source immediately. This is a really extraordinary achievement in a tiny object that weighs less than 0.1 g.

This quick overview from dolphins to bees seems to suggest that, based on the complexity of the behavior, some form of primary consciousness could be present in many species beyond humans. Let us now move further to the right along the x-axis, and cross the divide between the animate and the inanimate. First of all, let us consider a GPS. Listen to that persuasive voice telling you which is the best route to a secluded resort with greater precision than your partner does. What about your laptop, which never fails to beat you at chess? Not to mention those supercomputers such as Watson that can answer any question better than any human. There can be no doubt that these gadgets, which can produce language and calculations, would have given Descartes food for thought. Just imagine if he had met Alex the African Grey parrot and then encountered the supercomputer Deep Blue playing chess with Kasparov. At the very least, he would have been in a quandary, as his philosophical system basically assumed that the power to speak and calculate was an indication of the presence of consciousness. In spite of this, we are convinced that our GPS, our laptop, and Deep Blue are less endowed with consciousness than a parrot, an octopus, or a bee—indeed, most of us are convinced that they are completely unconscious. We would rate them at zero consciousness in our chart, just as we would rate headphones, calculators, and lawnmowers. But hold on a minute! Why do we think so? It often boils down to this: that we built them ourselves, we know exactly how they work, and we know that their impressive performance is due to speed of calculation and the respect of a series of basic rules (including learning rules) that we ourselves have imposed. Who is there to say that this makes them radically inferior to many animal species that show complex behaviors built in by evolution and natural selection? This is the problem with the consciousness/behavior relation: however appealing it may be, the mere fact that a behavior repertoire is complex and "cognitively sophisticated" is not sufficient to clinch the case for the presence of consciousness. Indeed, it isn't even a necessary condition. As we have already underscored in several occasions, it would be a serious error to deny consciousness to an unresponsive patient lying in pain in a hospital ward, or to a man happily dreaming in his bed. It is probably just as serious an error to deny consciousness to a dolphin that has opted to pass its existence watching bubbles of air rising through the water and is not going to tell us about what it feels like.

Brains

What about other objective criteria, the sheer mass of neurons? A natural expectation is that there should be some relation between the amount of brain tissue and the capacity for consciousness. Actually, we are so sure of the general value of this rule, that we identify the death of an individual with the death of all (or almost all) of his neurons, so it is worthwhile taking a moment to reflect on the relationship between the quantity of neurons and the capacity for consciousness in the inhabitants of the biological universe, particularly as the physical dimension of the brain can be measured quite accurately [250]. The size of the various brains in the mammalian world vary enormously; the sperm whale takes first place, weighing in at 7 kg, while at the end of the scale we find the hamster with a tiny brain that weighs just 1 g. In between there is the elephant with a respectable 5-kg brain, the dolphin with 1.5 kg, humans just below the dolphins at 1400 g, monkeys at 400 g, dogs at 80 g and parrots at 6 g [251]. These values cannot be said to be indicative of the extent of the animal's cognitive faculties, however. The dimension and weight of a brain primarily depend on the dimension and weight of the animal; larger animals need more and larger neurons, to control the basic functions of the host. An elephant will need many more receptors, sensory and motor neurons to control its immense surface (an elephant's skin can reach a dimension of 20 m²) and muscle mass (the trunk alone contains up to 100,000 muscles) than a hamster. Therefore, before thinking about the brain's dimensions in relation to the cognitive functions, the variable has to be somehow corrected for the size of the animal.

Comparative neuroanatomy has addressed this issue by using an index, known as the encephalization quotient (EQ), which is an approximate measure of relative brain size as defined by the ratio between the actual brain mass and the predicted brain mass of a given animal [252]. On average, in mammals the dimension of the neural system increases in relation to the size of the animal, following an exponential curve (with a power of approximately 0.66). Some species are collocated below this average curve and others above; the EQ quantifies the deviation from the average. The concept behind this exercise is that the excess neurons, the ones that are not strictly necessary for regulating the basic functions of the body, can be dedicated to the higher cognitive functions. In fact, when the EQ as opposed to the simple weight of the brain is adopted as the criterion, the ranking changes quite significantly. Humans shoot to the top with an EQ ratio of 6.5, followed by dolphins (5.5), chimpanzees (2.6), elephants (1.8), dogs (1.2), parrots (1), hamsters (0.6) and last the sperm whale with 0.26. This system of measurement has its limits—it is only applicable to mammals, it tends to penalize larger animals (like the sperm whale) and it does not take into consideration the number of neurons (which, of course, is an important factor in the weight of the brain). However, in spite of these shortcomings, it does provide a scale that is, at least intuitively, much more acceptable than that of the mere weight of the cerebral mass. So, could it be used as a reliable indicator of the capacity for consciousness in the animal kingdom? Probably not. Remember that the 20 billion neurons of our thalamocortical system are worth much, much more than the 70 billion neurons in the cerebellum. As we have seen, within the human brain, it is not the mass of neurons or their density that counts, but how they are organized. So, what is the effective weight for consciousness of the 250 billion neurons that constitute the elephant's brain? Just the 7 billion neurons in its cerebral cortex? Which are more important, the 15 billion neurons in the cortex of a fin whale or the 10 billion of the gorilla's cortex? The 150 million neurons in the cerebral cortex of a dog or the 500 million of the octopus' brain? Apart from some organizational aspects that are common to most beings, the neural cells, and their connectors often form different architectures in different species. The human nervous system is different to that of a dolphin, which is very different to that of a parrot, which in turn has little in common with the nervous system of a fish or a bee [253]. The octopus is a case apart; at least two-thirds of its neurons are decentralized in its tentacles. The bee contains about 800,000 nerve cells whose morphological and electrical heterogeneity rivals that of any neocortical neuron. These cells are assembled in highly non-linear feedback circuits whose density is up to 10 times higher than that of neocortex [254]. Is the bee's brain central complex, with its remarkable intricacy, more like the cerebellum or more like the cerebral cortex with respect to experience? When a bee navigates a maze, does it do so like when we consciously deliberate whether to turn right or left, or rather like when we play a well-learned piano piece in a seemingly non-conscious manner?

A Principled Approach

It would seem that both the functionalistic approach (which adopts behavior as a criterion) and the brain power-based approach (which relies on the number of neurons) leave much room for arbitrary choices. The alien consciousness-explorer visiting the planet, from the sky to the abyss, would get confused at some point. After all, a similar disorientation occurs to the neurologist visiting brain-injured patients armed with behavioral scales and brain scans. In the case of human injured brains, a principled approach turned out to be quite useful. Can a theory help in orienting ourselves, in guiding our practical decisions about the distribution of consciousness in the world?

To begin with, IIT can explain why both the functionalistic approach and the neuron-count may not work so well [255]. This is well illustrated by the two systems depicted in Figure 8.1. To the eye of an external observer, the two systems display the exact same behavior; that is, for the same inputs, the two networks will yield exactly the same outputs, they are functionally equivalent. If the external observer counts the number of elements (or neurons) that compose the two systems, he also realizes that the example on the right contains four times more neurons (38 vs 6) than the system on the left. Hence, by a purely external perspective, relying on observable behavior and brain size, he would be probably inclined to say that, if anything, the system on the right has a slight edge.

In the perspective of IIT, instead, the two physical systems could not be more different. The system on the left contains, between inputs and outputs, a core of positive Φ because there is a set of elements that are reciprocally connected through recurrent connections. The system on the right, instead, is a purely feed-forward network in which one layer feeds the next one without any recurrent causal interaction. In a feed-forward network, the input layer is always determined entirely by external inputs and the output layer does not affect the rest of the system, and the same is true recursively for the next layers downstream and upstream. This kind of system cannot make a difference to itself, it has no intrinsic cause–effect power and has $\Phi = 0$ [149]. According to IIT, then, such a feed-forward network completely lacks integration and does not exist intrinsically, for itself, but is a zombie, even if it performs quickly a range of tasks and even if it is larger.

The fact that any complex neural network with feedback circuits can be mapped (using many more neurons and connections) onto a purely feed-forward network in such a manner that the latter approximates or fully reproduces its input–output relationships is of capital importance. In the extreme case, a huge, purely feed-forward system able to

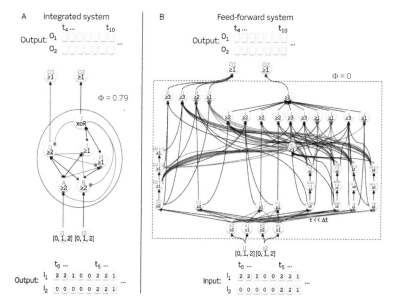

Figure 8.1 complicated, intelligent systems can be unconscious. (A) A strongly integrated system made of six elements (ABDHIJ) forms a complex with $\Phi = 0.76$. (B) Given many more elements ($n = 38$) and connections, it is possible to construct a feed-forward network implementing the same input–output function as the strongly integrated system in (A). However, in the feed-forward network, the input layer is always determined entirely by external inputs and the output layer does not affect the rest of the system; hence, neither layer can be part of a complex, and the same is true recursively for the next layers downstream and upstream. According to IIT, then, a feed-forward network does not exist intrinsically—for itself—but is a zombie—carrying out tasks unconsciously. Thus, despite the functional equivalence, the feed-forward system is unconscious, a "zombie" without phenomenological experience.

replicate the input-output behavior of the human brain would be behaviorally indistinguishable from us, yet it would have zero Φ and would thus be a "perfect" zombie [255]. Something along this direction may be already happening with present-day digital computers that, thanks to the exponential increase of computational power and memory capacity, can execute the appropriate algorithms to outperform us in many tasks. Feed-forward networks like those used in deep learning can label images, recognize animals, emotions through facial expressions, and much more. Last year, AlphaGo a computer program based on advanced deep-learning methods running on chips optimized for neural networks, has challenged the world Go top-ranked players [256]. Go is a popular board game, invented in China more than 2500 years ago, is much more complex than chess and was regarded by artificial intelligence experts as a hard problem. Not any more: AlphaGo has beaten all opponents including current world No.1 player, leaving astonished not only the Go community, but society at large.[1] However, this was only the beginning. AlphaGoZero, an updated algorithm using a method called reinforcement learning figured out how to play Go by itself, without the need for any human example, dataset, or intervention [257]. Learning from scratch, in only 40 days it became the best world player suggesting that the same approach could be transplanted from the game of Go to any other domain. Indeed, while this book is going to press, a generalization of AlphaGoZero, simply called AlphaZero, has been presented; AlphaZero learned on its own how to excel in three different board games, Go, chess, and shogi. Time will tell if the holy grail of artificial general intelligence is finally within reach. However, even if one day an updated version of these digital champions was to learn how to pass the Turing test it would not be conscious according to IIT, as long as it is organized like the system depicted on the right side of Figure 8.1.

What about a software that simulates in detail not just our behavior, but even the biophysics of neurons, synapses, and so on of the relevant portion of the human brain, such as the one imagined in Chapter 3? Functionalism would hold that it would be absolutely conscious, as in this case all the relevant functional roles within our brain, not just input–output relationships would have been replicated faithfully. According to IIT, however, this would be not justified, for the simple reason that the

---

1 An article published on January 5, 2017 in the *Wall Street Journal*, entitled "Humans Mourn Loss After Google Is Unmasked as China's Go Master", reported an interview with the No.1 ranking Go player Ke Jie stated: "After humanity spent thousands of years improving our tactics, computers tell us that humans are completely wrong ... I would go as far as to say not a single human has touched the edge of the truth of Go".

brain is real, but a simulation of the brain is virtual. Simulating a black hole, will not bend time and space. For the theory, consciousness is a fundamental property of physical systems, one that requires having real cause–effect power intrinsically. This goes along with our intuition that we would not feel comfortable to trade, even for a minute, our perishable brain for its eternal simulation. All these performances and computations would score o on the y-axis of our graph. Of course, for the computer that is running the simulation, which is as real as the brain, it is a different story. Here, everything depends on how elements, say transistors, are arranged. Current architectures would probably break down into mini-complexes with very low Φ, whereas future evolutions of current neuromorphic circuits [258], where the cause–effect power of the biological brain is emulated on a different substrate, may score much higher. The bottom line is that, according to IIT, it is not so much what a system does, but how it does it, that determines whether it is conscious.

In this perspective, things become much more interesting and unpredictable as we move back to the left on our graph to analyze the biological world. Here, evolutionary pressure may have naturally selected systems that carry on the same behavioral feats with less elements and more recurrent connections, due to space and energy constraint. Yet, neuronal properties and architectures may vary extremely, and together with Φ. Take again the cerebellum with its myriad of feed-forward circuits or the parallel unidirectional loops of the basal ganglia. Or consider our own thalamocortical system during NREM sleep, which turns into a largely feed-forward machine due to the breakdown of recurrent interactions brought about by bistable dynamics. We know how it feels to be such strange neuronal animals: as far as we can tell, it feels like nothing or close to nothing. What kind of neuronal animals are out there, beyond the walls of our skull?

It is true that neuro-anatomical and neurophysiological data for the incredibly variegated animal world are not as detailed as those available for the human species, but a genuinely theoretical approach can still offer a valid starting point to venture some predictions. For example, if a detailed analysis of the cerebral network formed by the 500 million neurons of the octopus were to demonstrate that they do not form an integrated system, but break down instead into a collection of small modules within each tentacle, we would have to conclude that, notwithstanding its agility, coordination, and predisposition for learning, the capacity for consciousness of the octopus would not be much greater than that of our cerebellum. The cephalopod can be tossed into the cooking pot with the same lack of qualms that the neurosurgeon throws the diseased cerebellum into the surgical waste bin. For now, however, we still do not know.

A similar line of reasoning could be applied to the brain of certain fish, which appear to have separate visual, tactile, gustative, and olfactory channels, each of which is able to regulate the fish's behavior autonomously. What would be the verdict in this case? It looks as if these brains are fragmented into a collection of parallel channels, similar to those of our basal ganglia, in which cases we should not worry much about their internal feelings.

What about the brains of our feathered friends? It is true that we sometimes use the term "bird brain" to indicate a person of little cognitive agility, but in point of fact the tiny cranium of the bird contains an extraordinarily well-developed cerebellum, much more sophisticated than the computer of a brand new airliner. However, it has not yet been resolved whether the other neurons are organized in a pattern similar to our basal ganglia or to that of the thalamocortical system [259], and as we have seen, this is an essential piece of the puzzle. If they are organized in a parallel feed-forward pattern similar to that of our basal ganglia loops, the words that Alex tweeted will be no more conscious than those spoken by SIRI or the GPS navigator. On the other hand, if uttered by something with an architecture more akin to the system depicted in Figure 8.1, those same words might be expressing the experiences and wishes of a tiny being endowed with a modicum of subjective experience.

Above and beyond architectures, differences in the biophysical properties of neurons may also play a very important role. For example, a recent study has shown that pyramidal neurons of the human neocortex have a membrane capacitance that is half the capacitance of rodent pyramidal neurons [260]. According to simulations, this difference has a major impact on signal transfer, by enhancing synaptic and action potential transmission, neuronal excitability, and possibly recurrent interactions. As we have seen in the previous chapter, where we have considered the effects of increased potassium conductance during sleep, small changes in intrinsic membrane properties may dramatically affect the strength and the nature of causal interactions among neurons. The field of comparative neurophysiology is in its infancy and many surprises lay ahead of us. In all cases, one should consider the possibility that even small deviations of the biophysical properties of neurons across species may affect the intrinsic cause–effect power of a system, and thus its Φ value, in substantial and surprising ways [253]. To evaluate this, observing neuroanatomy is not enough and in vivo measures must be adopted.

An Interesting Landscape

According to IIT, Φ can be graded. In us it may become higher as we grow from a baby to an adult whose brain has fully matured and becomes more functionally specialized. It can also increase and collapse when we are highly alert or drowsy, intoxicated by drugs or alcohol, or become demented in old age. Similarly, its values can vary largely within the animal kingdom, and even beyond, depending on how biological and physical systems are organized. A corollary of IIT that violates common intuitions is that even simple circuits can have a little bit of Φ and thus a minimal capacity for consciousness, provided that they are not purely feed-forward. By the same token, even when we fall in the deepest of NREM sleep, Φ is not going to be zero: when the thalamocortical system "disintegrates" due to bistability, it is likely to break down into many small complexes constituted of local groups of neurons linked by some recurrent causal interactions. What is it like to be an intrinsic entity with a low Φ value? How much should the absolute value of Φ matter for ethical concerns?

To try and address such questions properly, we need to wrap up our rudimentary TMS/EEG equipment, stow it in the basement and fast-forward to the future, trusting on the steady development of measurement techniques in neuroscience. It is conceivable that one day we will be able to systematically stimulate and record the brain at the appropriate spatial and temporal scale, moving closer to the exhaustive measure of Φ, as it was sketched in Chapter 5. For example, we could imagine the ability to stimulate neurons optogenetically, while simultaneously recording the firing activity of a population of neurons via two-photon calcium imaging to exhaustively assess its information capacity. We could, again, use optogenetics to temporarily deactivate specific connections in order to experimentally "partition" the brain and test for the irreducibility of its cause–effect repertoires. With a giant leap of imagination, we could envisage a universal probe that can read out the instantaneous values of Φ when aimed at any system, from the brain of a worm to that of a human. At this point, we could systematically compare how conscious we feel subjectively with the objective read-out of Φ and gradually become experts in matching our subjective state to the state of its physical substrate, like excellent wine tasters. We would appreciate this relationship while we are engaged in deep self-reflection, totally absorbed by a sunset, extremely tired, fighting to stay awake in front of the TV, drunk after a big night with friends, under sedation, waking up from deep sleep, from a strange dream, and so forth. Of course, we would not be able to experience and read out all possible levels of Φ. As we have already discussed, due to physical constraints in our brain (thresholds, non-linear amplifications, voltage dependent channels and so on), it is likely that during physiological adult life, Φ will jump in big steps from high to low values, and back. We may even learn that our own subjective judgement, which typically relies on introspection and memory, may not always be fully reliable when it comes to subtle gradations in the level of our own consciousness, especially when the level is low. In due time, however, it should be possible to establish rough calibration and a practical, conservative threshold of Φ or some related index such that nobody (including ourselves) ever reported that "there was something it was like to be us" when the read-out was below that value and another threshold above which some sort of experience was invariably present. For example, we could establish the typical value of Φ corresponding to when we are in deep sleep or anesthesia. Whatever that value may turn out to be, we will know that, from our own intrinsic perspective, that level of existence is nearly insignificant, meaning that it does not feel like much at all—very close to not existing at all. At his point, we could point the probe to the alien world outside of our brains and look at its landscape from a different perspective.

For all practical purposes, then, if we are able to establish that an octopus could never exceed the lower threshold of Φ, we could conclude that, whatever little amount of consciousness is in there, it does not matter either intrinsically or extrinsically—it will feel like so little that, compared with consciousness as we know it, it might as well feel like nothing. As a loose metaphor, consider temperature. While for us the difference between 0°C and 10°C matters, that between −260°C and −270°C matters much less—both are inconceivably cold. However, we might find instead that octopuses and parrots systematically score well above the lower threshold, or within the range of a 1-year-old human, or even within the range of our dreams. Whatever the answer, we will have, for the first time, a principled way of drawing a comparison between us, an octopus, a parrot, or the future version of AlphaZero. At the least, we could avoid gross mistakes—that is, to overlook a capacity for experience (experience, as we know it)—when we are forced to make choices in a world that is becoming more and more complicated.

We do not know its profile, but we suspect that the graph with some empirical measure of Φ on the y-axis may turn out to have an interesting and surprising shape—almost certainly neither the "all or nothing" distribution that Descartes proposed, nor the straight line endorsed by Montaigne. Indeed, the theory itself both enlarges and restricts the scope of what is conscious. It is likely that highly intelligent artifacts, such as supercomputers that may emulate and surpass our intelligence, may turn out to be unconscious, just like the cerebellum or the basal ganglia. Yet it is just as likely that a capacity for experience will be found in physical subtrates well beyond the human thalamocortical system, in entities that may not strike us as worth much in terms of behavior or intelligence, in places we did not expect—in the depths of the sea, in the sky, in an isolated bed in a long-term ward, and maybe one day, into the heart of a neuromorphic circuit. We may not yet know what it feels like to be in there, but we may infer that it feels like something.

CHAPTER 9

A UNIVERSE IN YOUR PALM

We look other people square in the eye, we shake their hand, touch their skin, but their brain is always well hidden away. Inaccessible. It is closed in a rigid box that protects it from mechanical injury, and also prevents us from coming to terms each day with the fact that this organ, too, is composed of matter (flesh, to put it bluntly); it has its own weight, smell, and a particular texture. If the central nervous system were exposed somewhere on the surface of our body, or if it were visible through a glass skull, we would be constantly faced with its paradoxes. As it is, only neurosurgeons have this privilege; each day they touch brains, manipulate them, stimulate them, cut away pieces. The brain has no nerves: it does not feel pain and so can be handled, while subjects are awake. Imagine what it must be like to stimulate the wet surface of the cortex with a clumsy bipolar electrode and hear the voice of the patient, from the other side of the green curtain, saying, "I see a light now." What it is like to suck up that same clammy matter with a sort of hoover, and hear it gurgle like crème caramel in a straw, when the owner of the brain is there, waiting for her epileptic focus to be removed? At the end of the first chapter, we left our student in the autopsy room, holding the brain of another human in his hand; unlike most neurosurgeons, he has had a lot of free time to ponder. At this point of the book, we step back into his shoes to share, in random order, some considerations with an existential flavor.

Extrinsic and Intrinsic

When the student was comparing the weight of the brain with the weight of the liver and of other organs, perhaps he felt a bit like Jacques Monod's alien researchers in their attempts to define the difference between animate and inanimate. This greyish mass that can see, suffer, and dream, at first glance does not seem to have anything special about it. The substance of experience is not wider, nor heavier. How can this object gain an intrinsic, subjective perspective? In that fateful moment, he did not search for an explanation of all the facets and possible contents of human experience; he just wanted to find a way to size-up a general capacity for consciousness in the physical world; perhaps not the best way, but a better one. Above all, he was driven by the instinct to touch, weigh, and measure.

After the shock in the morgue, the student returned to his studies, and devoured books and scientific articles. He understood that chains of neurons organized in multiple layers can carry out extremely complicated computations, such as detecting light waves of differing length, discriminating faces, grasping objects, and so on. He also came to the conclusion, that all these functions, however complicated they are, can be replicated by fast machines running sophisticated algorithms, without consciousness being there. He then left the library and the lecture rooms to join rounds in the ICU and neurological wards, where consciousness may fade, return, and hide disconnected from the world outside. Navigating through a jungle of drip-feeds, tubes, and respirators, he realized that even when the full technological arsenal of neuroscience is deployed, consciousness can escape, like the sea swirling through a fishing net. Surely, if subjective experience is not an illusion and has to do with the brain, the difference between consciousness and unconsciousness cannot hide in a detail. At the very least, it must be comparable with the difference between steam and ice, a change is the state of matter, as a physicist would say [261]. If we are unable to reliably detect this difference it must be because we are missing something fundamental. Perhaps the problem should be examined from a different perspective.

At this point, our student realized that the only way forward is to take a step back; forget the brain and start from the only thing we can know for certain, from the fundamental properties of our experience—consciousness exists, is highly informative, and is integrated. A minimal set of first principles, probably not the complete list, but enough to start a new kind of exploration through the physical world. A frantic expedition inside and outside the cranium, through the cortex, cerebellum, and basal ganglia, between sleep, dreams, anesthesia, and back again to the neurological ward, armed with a magnetic probe; an expedition that dared stretching to the realm of octopuses, parrots, crystals, and fast supercomputers. From all this, the student emerged dazed and confused. It had all been too quick, many important details were glossed over, the examples were not always a perfect fit, the measurements rough and certainly not as accurate as he would have wished. Despite this, he felt that he had a glimpse of what he was looking for.

In the first place, his initial intuition that something was missing was more than justified. A key challenge in appreciating what makes the brain so special when compared with other physical bodies was due to a fundamental misunderstanding. Now, it is clear that, while science has discovered how to measure many properties of natural objects—extension, mass, luminosity, temperature, and so on—one essential attribute, unity, has never been seriously considered, let alone measured. No attempts have been made at establishing an objective criterion by which to decide whether a given object is one integrated entity or an aggregate of smaller units. An object is usually defined as one entity when it has clear boundaries that distinguish it from its neighbors, when its pieces are well glued together or move in synchrony, when it has a volume, a weight that can be expressed as a number, or when it can be identified with a name. Thus, the property of "being one" has been attributed somewhat generously to objects in general, to galaxies, mountains, cities, biological structures, video-cameras, and many more. This is the origin of the misunderstanding—the gift of unity is given after a superficial examination from the extrinsic perspective, rather than from the intrinsic perspective of the system under consideration. The experiment with the camera is a perfect example of this. Looking at it from the outside, the camera appears as a single object, but the camera does not exist in and of itself, because within its sensor array differences do not make any difference. In fact, the function of the camera did not change when the sensor array was cut into millions of pieces; it was simply reduced to the single mechanisms of the individual photodiodes and nothing more. This experiment taught the student that establishing whether an object is a single entity is not easy, but it can be done. Only maxima of integrated information exist and the razor of Φ is merciless. Within the plastic case of the camera, individual photodiodes were all that existed.

When the student applies this new perspective to the organs that he had handled in the autopsy room, he sees them in a new light. The liver and the heart melt and shrink; the cerebellum and the basal ganglia disintegrate, just like the camera. Weak links and chains made of myriads of neurons break easily, splitting systems and peeling them down to their bones. Everything crumbles, except for an irreducible core within the thalamocortical system. Emerging from the morgue late at night, the student sees two fellows talking across the street. Within each brain there is a major thalamocortical complex—a maximally irreducible cause–effect structure with a high value of Φ. Because they are both talking and listening to each other, they also form a larger system with some positive level of Φ, but it is not maximally irreducible; the larger system has a value of Φ that is much less than that of each major complex it contains. Now, it is clear to the student that, by the intrinsic perspective, there is nothing it is like to be two people, let alone the 10 billion citizens of the world. He mentally probes other complicated objects and sees them dissolve into much lesser beings; mountains into heaps of sand; the supercomputer Watson into transistors; cities and buildings into aggregates of thermostats. Then, he turns toward the sky and, for a split second, sees the stars and the Milky Way dissolving as a heap of sand. He remembers a poem, one that is dear to many neuroscientists, one that he has found quoted in many books about the brain, and one that he finally understands it in all its power:

The brain is wider than the sky,
For, put them side by side,
The one the other will include
With ease, and you beside.

The brain is deeper than the sea,
For, hold them, blue to blue,
The one the other will absorb,
As sponges, buckets do.

The brain is just the weight of God,
For, lift them, pound for pound,
And they will differ, if they do,
As syllable from sound.

Perhaps, in a century or so, a scientist will fully demonstrate with formulas and measurements what a poet revealed with a delicate flick of the wrist, well over 100 years ago. Our student is not that scientist, nor a poet, but he feels inspired. If integrated information were like heat, the awake thalamocortical system would be as hot as the center of the sun;

if it were light, it would be brighter than any of the known stars; and if it were an extension, it would simply be the grandest. He sneaks back into the morgue and takes the brain in the palm of his hand. He is now moved to see the largest entity existing in the known universe, the most dense and intense, dressed in such modest clothing.

Actual and Potential

Now the student has another thought. In theory, measuring Φ requires assessing the repertoire of states that is available to a physical system *if* it were perturbed in all possible ways. Thus, consciousness, depends on the potential of the brain. However, the student reasons, I am conscious here and now, consciousness is the most actual thing there is. To be conscious, I don't need to explore the potential of my brain to establish the dimension of its repertoire of alternative states; this is bizarre! Then the student recalls that the definition of mass, which is the most actual property that a physical object possesses, is also given in potential, dispositional terms; the more mass a body has, the less its speed would change when it receives a force. Yet, it does not take a force to have a mass, the student thinks—a body does not need to calculate how its speed would change subject to a force, to have mass; nor does a brain need to compute its responses to perturbations to be conscious. Only if you want to *measure* mass, do you need to perturb the body with a force. The same is true for the brain. Practically, the capacity for consciousness could be assessed reliably by the perturbational complexity index: during the experiments, it was not enough to observe what the brain was doing, but one had to apply a magnetic perturbation to learn what it could do. Essentially, one had to shake the brain with a simple magnetic zap to reveal its capacity to unfold complex shapes from within. That was the only way to gauge intrinsic information as suggested by theoretical principles, and turned out to be quite effective. However, force and perturbations are to be applied only to measure the system's intrinsic properties from the exterior, but a system has its fundamental properties, whether they are measured or not. At each moment in time, what could have been is intrinsic to what is, just like mass is intrinsic to a body. So, the student ponders, a brain's evanescent and elusive consciousness may be as much or as little real as a body's mass, its most material aspect.

What if integrated information were, like mass, a fundamental property? In 1990, John Wheeler, a collaborator of Albert Einstein, Niels Bohr, and Enrico Fermi, coined the phrase "it from bit" [262]. For Wheeler, everything, every *it*—particles, magnetic fields, space, time—derives its function, its significance, and its very existence from a series of binary choices (*bit*), in other words, from information. This is certainly in line with IIT, but IIT is much more specific. First it emphasizes the essential relationship between information and causation. Causality is often interpreted as a reliable correlation between successively observed events. If we see that event A is regularly followed by event B, we deduce that A causes B. However, a complete definition of causality requires perturbations and a counter-check [263]. For instance, would effect B still have happened if, instead of imposing A, one had imposed perturbations C, D, E, and F? If it turned out that all perturbations result in effect B, we would begin to think that B was not so much caused by the preceding states, but rather that B was inevitable. In other words, the less a cause is specific (informative), the less it is a cause. Where information is diluted, causality is weak, and where there is the maximum possible information, causality is strongest. Crucially, according to IIT, the information that matters must also be integrated, that is irreducible—the physical substrate of consciousness is a maximum of irreducible cause–effect power. Seized by a burst of enthusiasm, the student imagines that if integrated information could be measured and expressed precisely like mass, the conscious brain would look like a giant black hole, bending space and time.

Outside and Inside

That image of a powerful black hole swirling in an empty universe throws a shadow over the whole subject. If the intrinsic prospective is the only one that counts, it follows that every consciousness is profoundly isolated. The notion that experience can be generated at any moment completely inside the walls of the skull seems to be correct, but implies hopeless solitude. The signals that come from the world outside are just meaningless electrical impulses and all the shapes of the world are woven within the unique loom of everyone's thalamocortical system. Thus, experience cannot be shared and each of us lives locked-in, a prisoner of a private garden generated within.

The student imagines a human brain that is forced to develop and grow in a vat. All the necessary nutrients and chemicals are added at the right time and in the right place, so that the genes can best express all that they know about the architecture of the nervous system. Over a period of weeks and months, the brain unfolds—it starts as a long tube that bends, swells, adds layers, eye buds, while neurons multiply at the astonishing pace of 250,000 elements/min [264], migrate, and stretch their axons far and wide. The axons wrap themselves in a thin layer of fat for insulation, and their ability to transmit becomes increasingly fast and efficient. This is all written down in the genetic instruction manual and is constructed faithfully to plan, up to the structural backbone of the thalamocortical system. However, since its first days, when it was a lump of cells, this brain received no input from the outside world, it never heard the blood rushing through the arteries of the uterus, far less its mother's heartbeat or her voice. It did not experience the suffocating grip of the birth channel, it did not yell as the first touch of air reached its lungs, it did not feel the warmth of its parent's embrace. It never went to school. It grew in total isolation, following its internal laws, those laws that have been determined by millions of years of slow and painful evolution. It becomes adult, but only because of the passage of time. Now what could this brain, whose sensory nerves have never transmitted any impulse, do? Maybe, it could dream. But of what? Perhaps, it would have only faded primordial dreams, maybe not even that.

According to IIT, consciousness develops with the repertoire of states that the brain can access, and the repertoire grows with its experience of the world. The thalamocortical system leaves the genetic factory in the form of a block of hyper-connected elements [265]. It is a very ductile block, ready to be carved in; in fact, brain circuits develop principally by removing existing connections, rather than by adding new ones. In the beginning, neurons are connected according to a basic plan, without much specificity and electrical activity looks as stereotypical as in deep NREM sleep or in the beating heart [266, 267]. Then, the core of innate connections is fine-tuned. Those that receive few impulses are gradually pruned away, allowing those that capture the events and coincidences of the external world, from the uterus to the great outside, to grow stronger [268]. From a very early age, babies are fascinated by cause–effect relationships [269]. They can spend hours pressing a switch to see if it causes an event (say, a given sound) in a reproducible manner, then they move to explore other switches and buttons to check all counterfactuals, to see whether they trigger different events. As these associations are incorporated into the neural circuits as synaptic connections, the intrinsic cause–effect repertoire grows. In time, the events captured by the brain become increasingly complex, the circuits become more specific, the number of possible internal states increases, and so does Φ.

The cause–effect repertoire is likely to grow at a very fast pace in these early exploratory stages of life [270], but may continue to grow throughout the person's lifespan, albeit at a significantly lower rate. In fact, it is not too hard to increase the number of possible states, even in an adult brain. For example, an adult can easily refine his knowledge of wines; with some training, a person who was initially unable to discriminate between red and white, gradually learns to appreciate different types of grapes, distinguish vineyards, and even the vintages. The neural circuits differentiate further and what before was identical becomes two, or many more, different states. This happens when we learn a new language, develop our taste in art, and every time we interact with other human beings. The number of possible conscious states available to an adult is so vast that adding another million or so through study, experience, and dedication is no great deal against the absolute value of Φ. However, from the early fetus to the grown-up human the difference might be substantial, maybe comparable with the one between sleep and wakefulness—nobody knows yet. What can be safely assumed is that, by selecting and pruning, the brain constructs an internal model of the external world; a model that may soon become so solid, general, and independent that the world can be dreamed from within. So, through dreaming, imagining, and creating, the internal repertoire continues to expand, even beyond the possibilities offered by the environment.

This string of reasoning, leads the student to two soothing conclusions. The first is that consciousness needs the world and other people to develop, but then it can grow and exist on its own; once external relations become internal, the universe exists from within. The second is that we might be not so lonely, after all. Our brain changes so much during our lifespan that the continuity of our identity may just rely on a collection of memories and beliefs. As long as these are similar enough from one moment to the next, the person can be said to stay the same. However, strip away your memories, beliefs, and self-reflections, abstract from your body and from the contingencies of senses, and you may share more with others than with our past or future selves. The medieval philosopher and mystic Meister Eckhart said:

> [. . .] if a man turns away from self and from all created things, then—to the extent that you do this—you will attain to oneness and blessedness in your soul's spark, which time and place never touched [. . .] [271]

Maybe, the student thinks, this is still our best shot toward immortality, surely better than simulating our brain's activity on a supercomputer. Coming relatively more down to earth, he remembers an old man he had seen coming day after day, for years, to the bedside of his wife. She had been severely stricken and was constantly unresponsive, but that did not seem to bother him at all. It was as if he felt that she was always there—in which brain, his or hers, probably did not matter.

Function and Experience

Like most of his peers, our student is deeply fascinated by computers and robots, ever more so by their amazing feats and speed. The same speed that when you Google something gives you the illusion of accessing the whole world at once. Only 20 years back it was perfectly normal to search for scientific articles on a library index, until it became possible to perform the first queries on a computer terminal; they seemed so fast at the time, but would feel unbearably slow today. Now, when our optic fiber connection slows down a bit, that extra second before a new page pops up seems an eternity, we feel the urge to click, double click, reload, or move the cursor to another link. We are conditioned by speed and action because we interact every day with machines that are becoming faster and faster.

The amount of information that is produced, transmitted, and stored in the world around us is growing at an unthinkable pace [272]. It is estimated that every year a few zettabyte (1 zettabyte = 10^{21} bytes) of new data is accumulated, which corresponds, more or less, to a pile of CD-ROMs five times higher than the distance from the earth to the moon. To put it in more human terms, this is the equivalent of giving each person living on earth today, 320 times the amount of information that was stored in the Library of Alexandria, which contained a copy of all books written before the 3rd century BC. It is difficult to convey the sheer magnitudes involved, but it is probably enough to consider that, in the year 2013 alone, an amount of information roughly equal to that previously accumulated by mankind was produced and stored, and that these figures are growing exponentially. In principle, and it may happen quite soon, everything under the sun will be quantified, digitized, and stored.

Analyzing this ocean of digital information, also known as big data, can be very useful in a wide range of domains, from matching the right people on dating sites to predicting epidemics, catastrophic meteorological events, diagnosing diseases, and much more. Since, for the human brain, crunching big data is inherently impossible, artificial intelligence is taking care of this. Every second, computers are applying algorithms to an unimaginable wealth of disparate data to infer probabilities—from the likelihood that an incoming email is spam to the probability that a given pattern of phone calls reflects an imminent terrorist attack. The secret of these machines is speed—extreme speed—so that they can be fed with lots of data on which to quickly discover patterns of correlations, make new predictions, and learn from their errors. The student is aware that much of mankind's future, from health care to the economy, will depend on these machines and on their algorithms, for better or for worse. He is confident that society will find ways to strike the right balance between a big data-driven prediction and a doctor's gut feeling about the prognosis of an individual patient, but he is disturbed by another vison—a giant grey cerebellum lurking over the planet like an alien vessel.

During his journey, he has had several occasions to note how often and how easily experience can dissociate from speed and performance. He saw that happening within his own head, where 70 billion neurons organized in feed-forward circuits predicted outcomes much better and much faster than he consciously did. His cerebellum could catch, without seeing, things that were absolutely out of reach for his thalamocortical system, such as a tennis ball flying at around 200 km/h. He understood that building an intrinsic perspective through integration takes time in the biological brain and that the price to pay for extreme speed is unconsciousness. He saw other people experiencing the most intense of dreams, while being disconnected and paralyzed, and others swiftly moving their fingers on the piano keyboard without even noticing. He met fully conscious LIS patients making superhuman efforts to slowly put together a word, one letter every few seconds, and compared them with Watson, which could access the equivalent of one million books (500 GB) every second and win Jeopardy, without being or feeling anything. Thus, he had learned that being and doing are two very different things, and that a functionalistic approach to consciousness can lead to fundamental misunderstandings.

Now, he sees how this issue may become paramount in the future. The whole world will be sampled, digitized, stored, and fed in yottabytes to supercomputers running machine-learning algorithms. However, this whole flood of information will remain extrinsic, quickly sweeping through the layers of a huge digital cerebellum running much of the world's business. We live together very well with our biological servants in the skull (we have evolved together), but how will it go with external, digital ones? Will they play the keyboard for us, and offer us more time and freedom to consciously enjoy the symphony of life? Or will the pressure for speed and performance prevail, thus making integrated, intrinsic information an even rarer specimen? In all cases, we shall be well prepared to appreciate experience, and its physical substrate, above and beyond performance, computations, predictive abilities, goal-directed behavior, and intelligence, so that we can take the time to enjoy and preserve it.

Periphery and Center

Scientific explanations of the mysteries of nature have given us the capacity to foresee, control, and manipulate the course of events, but they have also relentlessly stripped us of any illusions. First, the Copernican revolution ousted us from the center of the universe and relegated us to a tiny rock orbiting around a star, somewhere on the periphery of a galaxy in the middle of billions of other galaxies. Then came the theory of evolution, which shattered our dream of nobility—humanity was no longer the elect race, but just one of the multifarious outcomes of a game of blind chance and necessity. The essence of our lineage is reduced to a chain of molecules that is very similar to the chain of molecules that code for a mouse. Where will a scientific theory of consciousness land us?

Up to now, we have observed the universe with instruments that are only sensitive to mass, electrical charges, and energy. We have gazed on an immense empty space that contained enormous agglomerates—the stars and the planets—in comparison with which we are only a tiny mote of dust, a ridiculously small portion of all that exists. However, if the theory is correct and if one day we will be able to measure Φ with the same ease and precision with which, today, we can measure other physical quantities, the whole panorama may change radically. If we were able to measure integrated information—instead of mass, electrical charges, and energy—the planets and the galaxies would turn to grey dust and the universe would become even emptier and colder. Except for one place where we would see billions of new stars, glowing immense and bright. In this corner, the universe exists the most. Here, following millions of years of immense sacrifice, suffering, and courageous exploration, external relationships have become internal, ever richer and inseparable. Only here can light exist intrinsically, without the need for an external observer. Time will tell if another scientific revolution will return us to the center of our universe, naturally and on our merits. For now, like the astronaut who saw the earth lost in an icy space, the student is caught by a sense of wonder and deep affection. He would like to shield the weakest flames, the ones that struggle to awake and those that are fading, and decides that the best thing he can do is to explore, integrate and share, to understand the world, and let it exist a bit more.

REFERENCES

1. White, F. *The Overview Effect: Space Exploration and Human Evolution, Second Edition*, 2nd edn. Reston, VA: AIAA, 1998.
2. da Miller, G.A. *Psychology. The Science of Mental Life*. New York: Penguin Books.
3. Velmans, M. How to define consciousness: and how not to define consciousness. *J Conscious Stud* 2009; **16**: 139–56.
4. Jonkisz, J. Consciousness: a four-fold taxonomy. *J Conscious Stud* 2012; **19**: 55–82.
5. McGinn, C. Can we solve the mind–body problem? *Mind* 1989; **98**: 349–66.
6. Descartes, R., Cottingham, J., Stoothoff, R., and Murdoch, D. *The Philosophical Writings of Descartes*, vol. 1. Cambridge: Press Syndicate of Cambridge University Press, 1985.
7. Chalmers, D.J. *The Conscious Mind: In Search of a Fundamental Theory*. Revised edn. New York: Oxford University Press, 1997.
8. Thomas, N.J.T. Zombie killer. In: Hameroff, S.R., Kaszniak, A.W., and Scott, A.C. (eds). *Toward a Science of Consciousness*. Cambridge, MA: MIT Press, 1998.
9. Baker, S. *Final Jeopardy: Man vs. Machine and the Quest to Know Everything*. Boston: Houghton Mifflin Harcourt, 2011.
10. Turing, A.M. I.—Computing machinery and intelligence. *Mind* 1950; **LIX**: 433–60.
11. Ishiguro, H. Android science. In: Thrun, D.S., Brooks, D.R., Durrant-Whyte, D.H. (eds). *Robotics Research*. Berlin: Springer , 2007, pp. 118–27.
12. Searle, J.R. Minds, brains, and programs. *Behav Brain Sci* 1980; **3**: 417–24.
13. Koch, C. and Crick, F. The zombie within. *Nature* 2001; **411**: 893.
14. Townsend, J., Courchesne, E., Covington, J., *et al*. Spatial attention deficits in patients with acquired or developmental cerebellar abnormality. *J Neurosci Off J Soc Neurosci* 1999; **19**: 5632–43.
15. Schmahmann, J.D. Disorders of the cerebellum: ataxia, dysmetria of thought, and the cerebellar cognitive affective syndrome. *J Neuropsychiat Clin Neurosci* 2004; **16**: 367–78.
16. Singer, H.S. Tourette's syndrome: from behaviour to biology. *Lancet Neurol* 2005; **4**: 149–59.
17. Quiroga, R.Q., Reddy, L., Kreiman, G., *et al*. Invariant visual representation by single neurons in the human brain. *Nature* 2005; **435**: 1102–7.
18. Markram, H., Muller, E., Ramaswamy, S., *et al*. Reconstruction and simulation of neocortical microcircuitry. *Cell* 2015; **163**: 456–92.

19. Peduto, V.A., Silvetti, L., and Piga, M. [An anesthetized anesthesiologist tells his experience of waking up accidentally during the operation]. *Minerva Anestesiol* 1994; **60**: 1–5.

20. Sandin, R.H., Enlund, G., Samuelsson, P., et al. Awareness during anaesthesia: a prospective case study. *Lancet Lond* 2000; **355**: 707–11.

21. Mashour, G.A. and Avidan, M.S. Intraoperative awareness: controversies and non-controversies. *BJA Br J Anaesth* 2015; **115**: i20–6.

22. Lennmarken, C., Bildfors, K., Enlund, G., et al. Victims of awareness. *Acta Anaesthesiol Scand* 2002; **46**: 229–31.

23. Leslie, K., Chan, M.T.V., Myles, P.S., et al. Posttraumatic stress disorder in aware patients from the B-aware trial. *Anesth Analg* 2010; **110**: 823–8.

24. Cook, T.M., Andrade, J., Bogod, D.G., et al. 5th National Audit Project (NAP5) on accidental awareness during general anaesthesia: patient experiences, human factors, sedation, consent, and medicolegal issues. *Br J Anaesth* 2014; **113**: 560–74.

25. Aranake, A., Gradwohl, S., Ben-Abdallah, A., et al. Increased risk of intraoperative awareness in patients with a history of awareness. *Anesthesiology* 2013; **119**: 1275–83.

26. Sanders, R.D., Tononi, G., Laureys, S., et al. Unresponsiveness ≠ unconsciousness. *Anesthesiology* 2012; **116**: 946–59.

27. Russell, I.F. Comparison of wakefulness with two anaesthetic regimens. Total i.v. balanced anaesthesia. *Br J Anaesth* 1986; **58**: 965–8.

28. Pandit, J.J., Russell, I.F., and Wang, M. Interpretations of responses using the isolated forearm technique in general anaesthesia: a debate. *Br J Anaesth* 2015; **115**(Suppl. 1): i32–45.

29. Perouansky, M. and Pearce, R.A. How we recall (or don't): the hippocampal memory machine and anesthetic amnesia. *Can J Anaesth* 2011; **58**: 157–66.

30. Posner, J.B., Saper, C.B., Schiff, N., et al. *Plum and Posner's Diagnosis of Stupor and Coma*, 4th edn. Oxford: Oxford University Press, 2007.

31. Brown, E.N., Lydic, R., and Schiff, N.D. General anesthesia, sleep, and coma. *N Engl J Med* 2010; **363**: 2638–50.

32. Ibsen, B. Treatment of respiratory complications in poliomyelitis; the anesthetist's viewpoint. *Dan Med Bull* 1954; **1**: 9–12.

33. Berthelsen, P.G. Manual positive pressure ventilation and the Copenhagen Poliomyelitis Epidemic 1952: an attempt at setting the record straight. *Acta Anaesthesiol Scand* 2014; **58**(5): 503–7.

34. Laureys, S. Science and society: death, unconsciousness and the brain. *Nat Rev Neurosci* 2005; **6**: 899–909.

35. A definition of irreversible coma. Report of the Ad Hoc Committee of the Harvard Medical School to Examine the Definition of Brain Death. *JAMA* 1968; **205**: 337–40.

36. Giacino, J.T., Fins, J.J., Laureys, S., et al. Disorders of consciousness after acquired brain injury: the state of the science. *Nat Rev Neurol* 2014; **10**: 99–114.

37. Fins, J.J. *Rights Come to Mind: Brain Injury, Ethics, and the Struggle for Consciousness.* New York, NY: Cambridge University Press, 2015.
38. Laureys, S. The neural correlate of (un)awareness: lessons from the vegetative state. *Trends Cogn Sci* 2005; **9**: 556–9.
39. Jennett, B. and Plum, F. Persistent vegetative state after brain damage. A syndrome in search of a name. *Lancet Lond Engl* 1972; **1**: 734–7.
40. Laureys, S., Celesia, G.G., Cohadon, F., *et al.* Unresponsive wakefulness syndrome: a new name for the vegetative state or apallic syndrome. *BMC Med* 2010; **8**: 68.
41. León-Carrión, J., van Eeckhout, P., and Domínguez-Morales, M.D.R. The locked-in syndrome: a syndrome looking for a therapy. *Brain Inj* 2002; **16**: 555–69.
42. Laureys, S., Pellas, F., Van Eeckhout, P., *et al.* The locked-in syndrome: what is it like to be conscious but paralyzed and voiceless? *Prog Brain Res* 2005; **150**: 495–511.
43. Bauby, J.-D. *The Diving Bell and the Butterfly: A Memoir of Life in Death.* Princeton, NJ: Vintage, 1998.
44. Coghlan, P. *In the Blink of an Eye.* CreateSpace Independent Publishing Platform, 2013.
45. Tavalaro, J. and Tayson, R. *Look Up for Yes.* New York: Penguin USA, 1998.
46. Bruno, M.-A., Bernheim, J.L., Ledoux, D., *et al.* A survey on self-assessed well-being in a cohort of chronic locked-in syndrome patients: happy majority, miserable minority. *BMJ Open* 2011; **1**: e000039.
47. Bauer, G., Gerstenbrand, F., and Rumpl, E. Varieties of the locked-in syndrome. *J Neurol* 1979; **221**: 77–91.
48. Giacino, J. and Whyte, J. The vegetative and minimally conscious states: current knowledge and remaining questions. *J Head Trauma Rehabil* 2005; **20**: 30–50.
49. Giacino, J.T. and Kalmar, K. The vegetative and minimally conscious states: a comparison . . . *J Head Trauma Rehabil* 1997; **12**(4): 36–51.
50. Fins, J.J., Schiff, N.D., and Foley, K.M. Late recovery from the minimally conscious state: ethical and policy implications. *Neurology* 2007; **68**: 304–7.
51. Andrews, K., Murphy, L., Munday, R., *et al.* Misdiagnosis of the vegetative state: retrospective study in a rehabilitation unit. *Br Med J* 1996; **313**: 13–6.
52. Majerus, S., Gill-Thwaites, H., Andrews, K., *et al.* Behavioral evaluation of consciousness in severe brain damage. *Prog Brain Res* 2005; **150**: 397–413.
53. Schnakers, C., Vanhaudenhuyse, A., Giacino, J., *et al.* Diagnostic accuracy of the vegetative and minimally conscious state: clinical consensus versus standardized neurobehavioral assessment. *BMC Neurol* 2009; **9**: 35.
54. Strauss, D.J., Ashwal, S., Day, S.M., *et al.* Life expectancy of children in vegetative and minimally conscious states. *Pediatr Neurol* 2000; **23**: 312–19.
55. Giacino, J.T., Kalmar, K., and Whyte, J. The JFK Coma Recovery Scale-Revised: measurement characteristics and diagnostic utility. *Arch Phys Med Rehabil* 2004; **85**: 2020–9.

56. Bodien, Y.G., Carlowicz, C.A., Chatelle, C., *et al.* Sensitivity and specificity of the Coma Recovery Scale--Revised total score in detection of conscious awareness. *Arch Phys Med Rehabil* 2016; **97**: 490–2.e1.

57. Hayashi, H. and Kato, S. Total manifestations of amyotrophic lateral sclerosis. ALS in the totally locked-in state. *J Neurol Sci* 1989; **93**: 19–35.

58. Ragazzoni, A., Grippo, A., Tozzi, F., *et al.* Event-related potentials in patients with total locked-in state due to fulminant Guillain–Barré syndrome. *Int J Psychophysiol Off J Int Organ Psychophysiol* 2000; **37**: 99–109.

59. Cairns, H., Oldfield, R.C., Pennybacker, J.B., *et al.* Akinetic mutism with an epidermoid cyst of the 3rd ventricle. *Brain* 1941; **64**: 273–90.

60. Németh, G., Hegedüs, K., and Molnár, L. Akinetic mutism associated with bicingular lesions: clinicopathological and functional anatomical correlates. *Eur Arch Psychiatry Neurol Sci* 1988; **237**: 218–22.

61. Jang, S.H. and Kwon, H.G. Akinetic mutism in a patient with mild traumatic brain injury: a diffusion tensor tractography study. *Brain Inj* 2017: 1–5.

62. Boly, M., Coleman, M.R., Davis, M.H., *et al.* When thoughts become action: an fMRI paradigm to study volitional brain activity in non-communicative brain injured patients. *NeuroImage* 2007; **36**: 979–92.

63. Owen, A.M., Coleman, M.R., Boly, M., *et al.* Detecting awareness in the vegetative state. *Science* 2006; **313**: 1402.

64. Owen, A. *Into the Gray Zone: A Neuroscientist Explores the Border Between Life and Death.* New York, NY: Scribner, 2017.

65. Naci, L., Cusack, R., Anello, M., *et al.* A common neural code for similar conscious experiences in different individuals. *Proc Natl Acad Sci* 2014; **111**: 14277–82.

66. Monti, M.M., Vanhaudenhuyse, A., Coleman, M.R., *et al.* Willful modulation of brain activity in disorders of consciousness. *N Engl J Med* 2010; **362**: 579–89.

67. Fernández-Espejo, D. and Owen, A.M. Detecting awareness after severe brain injury. *Nat Rev Neurosci* 2013; **14**: 801–9.

68. Bayne, T., Hohwy, J., and Owen, A.M. Reforming the taxonomy in disorders of consciousness. *Ann Neurol* 2017; **82**(6): 866–72.

69. Bardin, J.C., Fins, J.J., Katz, D.I., *et al.* Dissociations between behavioural and functional magnetic resonance imaging-based evaluations of cognitive function after brain injury. *Brain J Neurol* 2011; **134**: 769–82.

70. Sutton, S., Braren, M., Zubin, J., *et al.* Evoked-potential correlates of stimulus uncertainty. *Science* 1965; **150**: 1187–8.

71. Bekinschtein, T.A., Dehaene, S., Rohaut, B., *et al.* Neural signature of the conscious processing of auditory regularities. *Proc Natl Acad Sci U S A* 2009; **106**: 1672–7.

72. King, J.R., Faugeras, F., Gramfort, A., *et al.* Single-trial decoding of auditory novelty responses facilitates the detection of residual consciousness. *NeuroImage* 2013; **83**: 726–38.

73. Faugeras, F., Rohaut, B., Weiss, N., et al. Probing consciousness with event-related potentials in the vegetative state. Neurology 2011; **77**: 264–8.

74. Dehaene, S. and Changeux, J.-P. Experimental and theoretical approaches to conscious processing. Neuron 2011; **70**: 200–27.

75. Dehaene, S. Consciousness and the Brain: Deciphering How the Brain Codes Our Thoughts. New York, NY: Viking, 2014.

76. Sitt, J.D., King, J.-R., El Karoui, I., et al. Large scale screening of neural signatures of consciousness in patients in a vegetative or minimally conscious state. Brain J Neurol 2014; **137**: 2258–70.

77. Melloni, L., Schwiedrzik, C.M., Müller, N., et al. Expectations change the signatures and timing of electrophysiological correlates of perceptual awareness. J Neurosci Off J Soc Neurosci 2011; **31**: 1386–96.

78. Aru, J., Bachmann, T., Singer, W., et al. Distilling the neural correlates of consciousness. Neurosci Biobehav Rev 2012; **36**: 737–46.

79. Pitts, M.A., Metzler, S., and Hillyard, S.A. Isolating neural correlates of conscious perception from neural correlates of reporting one's perception. Front Psychol 2014; **8**(5): 1078.

80. Pitts, M.A., Padwal, J., Fennelly, D., et al. Gamma band activity and the P3 reflect post-perceptual processes, not visual awareness. NeuroImage 2014; **101**: 337–50.

81. Koulack, D. Effects of somatosensory stimulation on dream content. Arch Gen Psychiatry 1969; **20**: 718–25.

82. Nir, Y. and Tononi, G. Dreaming and the brain: from phenomenology to neurophysiology. Trends Cogn Sci 2010; **14**: 88–100.

83. Hejja, P. and Galloon, S. A consideration of ketamine dreams. Can Anaesth Soc J 1975; **22**: 100–5.

84. Sullivan, P.R. Contentless consciousness and information-processing theories of mind. Philos Psychiat Psychol 1995; **2**: 51–9.

85. James, W. The Principles of Psychology, vol. 1. Mineola, NY: Dover Publications, 1950, 273.

86. Gosseries, O., Di, H., Laureys, S., et al. Measuring consciousness in severely damaged brains. Annu Rev Neurosci 2014; **37**: 457–78.

87. Koch, C., Massimini, M., Boly, M., et al. Neural correlates of consciousness: progress and problems. Nat Rev Neurosci 2016; **17**: 307–21.

88. Destexhe, A., Contreras, D., and Steriade, M. Spatiotemporal analysis of local field potentials and unit discharges in cat cerebral cortex during natural wake and sleep states. J Neurosci 1999; **19**: 4595–608.

89. Steriade, M., Timofeev, I., and Grenier, F. Natural waking and sleep states: a view from inside neocortical neurons. J Neurophysiol 2001; **85**: 1969–85.

90. DeSalvo, M.N., Schridde, U., Mishra, A.M., et al. Focal BOLD fMRI changes in bicuculline-induced tonic-clonic seizures in the rat. NeuroImage 2010; **50**: 902–9.

91. Stender, J., Gosseries, O., Bruno, M.-A., *et al.* Diagnostic precision of PET imaging and functional MRI in disorders of consciousness: a clinical validation study. *Lancet Lond Engl* 2014; **384**: 514–22.

92. Laureys, S., Antoine, S., Boly, M., *et al.* Brain function in the vegetative state. *Acta Neurol Belg* 2002; **102**: 177–85.

93. Frässle, S., Sommer, J., Jansen, A., *et al.* Binocular rivalry: frontal activity relates to introspection and action but not to perception. *J Neurosci Off J Soc Neurosci* 2014; **34**: 1738–47.

94. Noy, N., Bickel, S., Zion-Golumbic, E., *et al.* Ignition's glow: ultra-fast spread of global cortical activity accompanying local "ignitions" in visual cortex during conscious visual perception. *Conscious Cogn* 2015; **35**: 206–24.

95. Hebb, D.O. and Penfield, W. Human behavior after extensive bilateral removal from the frontal lobes. *Arch Neurol Psychiatry* 1940; **44**: 421–38.

96. Fulton, J.F. *Functional Localization in Relation to Frontal Lobotomy.* Oxford: Oxford University Press, 1949.

97. Brickner, R.M. Brain of patient A after bilateral frontal lobectomy; status of frontal-lobe problem. *AMA Arch Neurol Psychiatry* 1952; **68**: 293–313.

98. Mataró, M., Jurado, M.A., García-Sánchez, C., *et al.* Long-term effects of bilateral frontal brain lesion: 60 years after injury with an iron bar. *Arch Neurol* 2001; **58**: 1139–42.

99. Markowitsch, H.J. and Kessler, J. Massive impairment in executive functions with partial preservation of other cognitive functions: the case of a young patient with severe degeneration of the prefrontal cortex. *Exp Brain Res* 2000; **133**: 94–102.

100. Tsuchiya, N., Wilke, M., Frässle, S., *et al.* No-report paradigms: extracting the true neural correlates of consciousness. *Trends Cogn Sci* 2015; **19**: 757–70.

101. Siclari, F., Baird, B., Perogamvros, L., *et al.* The neural correlates of dreaming. *Nat Neurosci* 2017, **20**(6): 872–8.

102. Vanhaudenhuyse, A., Noirhomme, Q., Tshibanda, L.J.-F., *et al.* Default network connectivity reflects the level of consciousness in non-communicative brain-damaged patients. *Brain* 2010; **133**: 161–71.

103. Crick, F. and Koch, C. Some reflections on visual awareness. *Cold Spring Harb Symp Quant Biol* 1990; **55**: 953–62.

104. Fries, P., Roelfsema, P.R., Engel, A.K., *et al.* Synchronization of oscillatory responses in visual cortex correlates with perception in interocular rivalry. *Proc Natl Acad Sci U S A* 1997; **94**: 12699–704.

105. Rodriguez, E., George, N., Lachaux, J.P., *et al.* Perception's shadow: long-distance synchronization of human brain activity. *Nature* 1999; **397**: 430–3.

106. Singer W. Neuronal synchrony: a versatile code for the definition of relations? *Neuron* 1999; **24**: 49–65.

107. King, J.-R., Sitt, J.D., Faugeras, F., *et al.* Information sharing in the brain indexes consciousness in noncommunicative patients. *Curr Biol CB* 2013; **23**: 1914–19.

108. Chennu, S., Finoia, P., Kamau, E., *et al*. Spectral signatures of reorganised brain networks in disorders of consciousness. *PLoS Comput Biol* 2014; **10**: e1003887.

109. Supp, G.G., Siegel, M., Hipp, J.F., *et al*. Cortical hypersynchrony predicts breakdown of sensory processing during loss of consciousness. *Curr Biol CB* 2011; **21**: 1988–93.

110. Pockett, S. and Holmes, M.D. Intracranial EEG power spectra and phase synchrony during consciousness and unconsciousness. *Conscious Cogn* 2009; **18**: 1049–55.

111. Arthuis, M., Valton, L., Régis, J., *et al*. Impaired consciousness during temporal lobe seizures is related to increased long-distance cortical-subcortical synchronization. *Brain J Neurol* 2009; **132**: 2091–101.

112. Berger, H. Über das Elektrenkephalogramm des Menschen. *Arch Für Psychiatr Nervenkrankh* 1933; **99**: 555–74.

113. Steriade, M. Corticothalamic resonance, states of vigilance and mentation. *Neuroscience* 2000; **101**: 243–76.

114. Kales, A., Rechtschaffen, A., University of California, Los Angeles *et al*. (eds) *A Manual of Standardized Terminology, Techniques and Scoring System for Sleep Stages of Human Subjects*. Rechtschaffen, A. and Kales, A. (eds). Bethesda, MD: U. S. National Institute of Neurological Diseases and Blindness, Neurological Information Network, 1968.

115. McNamara, P., Johnson, P., McLaren, D., *et al*. REM and NREM sleep mentation. *Int Rev Neurobiol* 2010; **92**: 69–86.

116. Lewis, L.D., Weiner, V.S., Mukamel, E.A., *et al*. Rapid fragmentation of neuronal networks at the onset of propofol-induced unconsciousness. *Proc Natl Acad Sci U S A* 2012; **109**: E3377–86.

117. Ní Mhuircheartaigh, R., Warnaby, C., Rogers, R., *et al*. Slow-wave activity saturation and thalamocortical isolation during propofol anesthesia in humans. *Sci Transl Med* 2013; **5**: 208ra148.

118. Schiff, N.D., Nauvel, T., and Victor, J.D. Large-scale brain dynamics in disorders of consciousness. *Curr Opin Neurobiol* 2014; **25**: 7–14.

119. Forgacs, P.B., Conte, M.M., Fridman, E.A., *et al*. Preservation of electroencephalographic organization in patients with impaired consciousness and imaging-based evidence of command-following. *Ann Neurol* 2014; **76**: 869–79.

120. Westmoreland, B.F., Klass, D.W., Sharbrough, F.W., *et al*. Alpha-coma. Electroencephalographic, clinical, pathologic, and etiologic correlations. *Arch Neurol* 1975; **32**: 713–18.

121. Wikler, A. Pharmacologic dissociation of behavior and EEG "sleep patterns" in dogs; morphine, n-allylnormorphine, and atropine. *Proc Soc Exp Biol Med Soc Exp Biol Med N Y N* 1952; **79**: 261–5.

122. Bradley, P.B. The effect of atropine and related drugs on the EEG and behaviour. *Prog Brain Res* 1968; **28**: 3–13.

123. Gökyiğit, A. and Calişkan, A. Diffuse spike-wave status of 9-year duration without behavioral change or intellectual decline. *Epilepsia* 1995; **36**: 210–13.

124. Vuilleumier, P., Assal, F., Blanke, O., *et al.* Distinct behavioral and EEG topographic correlates of loss of consciousness in absences. *Epilepsia* 2000; **41**: 687–93.

125. Nobili, L., De Gennaro, L., Proserpio, P., *et al.* Local aspects of sleep: observations from intracerebral recordings in humans. *Prog Brain Res* 2012; **199**: 219–32.

126. Herculano-Houzel, S. The remarkable, yet not extraordinary, human brain as a scaled-up primate brain and its associated cost. *Proc Natl Acad Sci U S A* 2012; **109**(Suppl. 1): 10661–8.

127. Glickstein, M. and Doron, K. Cerebellum: connections and functions. *Cerebellum Lond Engl* 2008; **7**: 589–94.

128. Glickstein, M. What does the cerebellum really do? *Curr Biol CB* 2007; **17**: R824–7.

129. Palesi, F., Tournier, J.-D., Calamante, F., *et al.* Contralateral cerebello-thalamo-cortical pathways with prominent involvement of associative areas in humans in vivo. *Brain Struct Funct* 2015; **220**: 3369–84.

130. Boyd, C.A. Cerebellar agenesis revisited. *Brain* 2010; **133**: 941–4.

131. Lemon, R.N. and Edgley, S.A. Life without a cerebellum. *Brain* 2010; **133**: 652–4.

132. Yu, F., Jiang, Q., Sun, X., *et al.* A new case of complete primary cerebellar agenesis: clinical and imaging findings in a living patient. *Brain J Neurol* 2015; **138**: e353.

133. Siclari, F., LaRocque, J.J., Postle, B.R., *et al.* Assessing sleep consciousness within subjects using a serial awakening paradigm. *Front Psychol* 2013; **4**: 542.

134. Timofeev, I., Grenier, F., and Steriade, M. Disfacilitation and active inhibition in the neocortex during the natural sleep-wake cycle: an intracellular study. *Proc Natl Acad Sci U S A* 2001; **98**: 1924–9.

135. Compte, A., Sanchez-Vives, M.V., McCormick, D.A., *et al.* Cellular and network mechanisms of slow oscillatory activity (<1 Hz) and wave propagations in a cortical network model. *J Neurophysiol* 2003; **89**: 2707–25.

136. Aserinsky, E. and Kleitman, N. Regularly occurring periods of eye motility, and concomitant phenomena, during sleep. *Science* 1953; **118**: 273–4.

137. Stickgold, R., Malia, A., Fosse, R., *et al.* Brain-mind states: I. Longitudinal field study of sleep/wake factors influencing mentation report length. *Sleep* 2001; **24**: 171–9.

138. Hobson, J.A., Pace-Schott, E.F., Stickgold, R. Dreaming and the brain: toward a cognitive neuroscience of conscious states. *Behav Brain Sci* 2000; **23**: 793–842; discussion 904–1121.

139. Thiele, A., Henning, P., Kubischik, M., *et al.* Neural mechanisms of saccadic suppression. *Science* 2002; **295**: 2460–2.

140. Floyer-Lea, A. and Matthews, P.M. Changing brain networks for visuomotor control with increased movement automaticity. *J Neurophysiol* 2004; **92**: 2405–12.

141. Schiff, N.D. Recovery of consciousness after brain injury: a mesocircuit hypothesis. *Trends Neurosci* 2010; **33**: 1–9.

142. Straussberg, R., Shorer, Z., Weitz, R., *et al.* Familial infantile bilateral striatal necrosis: clinical features and response to biotin treatment. *Neurology* 2002; **59**: 983–9.

143. Caparros-Lefebvre, D., Destée, A. and Petit, H. Late onset familial dystonia: could mitochondrial deficits induce a diffuse lesioning process of the whole basal ganglia system? *J Neurol Neurosurg Psychiatry* 1997; **63**: 196–203.

144. Moruzzi, G. and Magoun, H.W. Brain stem reticular formation and activation of the EEG. *Electroencephalogr Clin Neurophysiol* 1949; **1**: 455–73.

145. Gazzaniga, M.S. The split-brain: rooting consciousness in biology. *Proc Natl Acad Sci U S A* 2014; **111**: 18093–4.

146. Bachmann, T. *Microgenetic Approach to the Conscious Mind.* Amsterdam: John Benjamins Publishing Company, 2000.

147. Tononi, G. An information integration theory of consciousness. *BMC Neurosci* 2004; **5**: 42.

148. Tononi, G., Boly, M., Massimini, M., *et al.* Integrated information theory: from consciousness to its physical substrate. *Nat Rev Neurosci* 2016; **17**: 450–61.

149. Oizumi, M., Albantakis, L., and Tononi, G. From the phenomenology to the mechanisms of consciousness: Integrated Information Theory 3.0. *PLoS Comput Biol* 2014; **10**: e1003588.

150. *BSTJ : A Mathematical Theory of Communication (Shannon, C.E.).*, 1948.

151. Sperry, R.W. Cerebral organization and behavior: the split brain behaves in many respects like two separate brains, providing new research possibilities. *Science* 1961; **133**: 1749–57.

152. Levisohn, L., Cronin-Golomb, A., and Schmahmann, J.D. Neuropsychological consequences of cerebellar tumour resection in children: cerebellar cognitive affective syndrome in a paediatric population. *Brain J Neurol* 2000; **123**(Pt 5): 1041–50.

153. Oscarsson, O. Functional units of the cerebellum—sagittal zones and microzones. *Trends Neurosci* 1979; **2**: 143–5.

154. Apps, R. and Garwicz, M. Anatomical and physiological foundations of cerebellar information processing. *Nat Rev Neurosci* 2005; **6**(4): 297–311.

155. Martin, T.A., Keating, J.G., Goodkin, H.P., *et al.* Throwing while looking through prisms. I. Focal olivocerebellar lesions impair adaptation. *Brain J Neurol* 1996; **119**(Pt 4): 1183–98.

156. Brunel, N., Hakim, V., Isope, P., *et al.* Optimal information storage and the distribution of synaptic weights: perceptron versus Purkinje cell. *Neuron* 2004; **43**: 745–57.

157. NIH Launches the Human Connectome Project to Unravel the Brain's Connections. *Natl Inst Health NIH* 2015. https://www.nih.gov/news-events/news-releases/nih-launches-human-connectome-project-unravel-brains-connections [accessed 18 January 2018].

158. Jarrell, T.A., Wang, Y., Bloniarz, A.E., *et al.* The connectome of a decision-making neural network. *Science* 2012; **337**: 437–44.

159. Bartels, A. and Zeki, S. The chronoarchitecture of the cerebral cortex. *Philos Trans R Soc Lond B Biol Sci* 2005; **360**: 733–50.

160. Van Essen, D.C. Cartography and connectomes. *Neuron* 2013; **80**: 775–90.

161. Caspers, S., Eickhoff, S.B., Zilles, K., *et al.* Microstructural grey matter parcellation and its relevance for connectome analyses. *NeuroImage* 2013; **80**: 18–26.

162. Ding, S.-L., Royall, J.J., Sunkin, S.M., *et al.* Comprehensive cellular-resolution atlas of the adult human brain. *J Comp Neurol* 2016; **524**: 3127–481.

163. Hill, S. and Tononi, G. Modeling sleep and wakefulness in the thalamocortical system. *J Neurophysiol* 2005; **93**: 1671–98.

164. Jirsa, V.K., Sporns, O., Breakspear, M., *et al.* Towards the virtual brain: network modeling of the intact and the damaged brain. *Arch Ital Biol* 2010; **148**: 189–205.

165. Deco, G., Tononi, G., Boly, M., *et al.* Rethinking segregation and integration: contributions of whole-brain modelling. *Nat Rev Neurosci* 2015; **16**: 430–9.

166. Amunts, K., Ebell, C., Muller, J., *et al.* The Human Brain Project: creating a European research infrastructure to decode the human brain. *Neuron* 2016; **92**: 574–81.

167. Friston, K.J. Modalities, modes, and models in functional neuroimaging. *Science* 2009; **326**: 399–403.

168. Bullmore, E. and Sporns, O. Complex brain networks: graph theoretical analysis of structural and functional systems. *Nat Rev Neurosci* 2009; **10**: 186–98.

169. Schiff, N., Ribary, U., Plum, F., *et al.* Words without mind. *J Cogn Neurosci* 1999; **11**: 650–6.

170. Stace, W.T. *Mysticism and Philosophy.* Los Angeles: Jeremy Tercher, 1987.

171. Jain, S.K., Sundar, I.V., Sharma, V., *et al.* Bilateral large traumatic basal ganglia haemorrhage in a conscious adult: a rare case report. *Brain Inj* 2013; **27**: 500–3.

172. Alexander, G.E., DeLong, M.R., and Strick, P.L. Parallel organization of functionally segregated circuits linking basal ganglia and cortex. *Annu Rev Neurosci* 1986; **9**: 357–81.

173. McHaffie, J.G., Stanford, T.R., Stein, B.E., *et al.* Subcortical loops through the basal ganglia. *Trends Neurosci* 2005; **28**: 401–7.

174. Parvizi, J. and Damasio, A. Consciousness and the brainstem. *Cognition* 2001; **79**: 135–60.

175. Libet, B. *Mind Time: The Temporal Factor in Consciousness.* Cambridge, MA: Harvard University Press, 1634.

176. Eagleman, D.M. and Sejnowski, T.J. Motion integration and postdiction in visual awareness. *Science* 2000; **287**: 2036–8.

177. Libet, B. Brain stimulation in the study of neuronal functions for conscious sensory experiences. *Hum Neurobiol* 1982; **1**: 235–42.

178. Sergent, C., Baillet, S., and Dehaene, S. Timing of the brain events underlying access to consciousness during the attentional blink. *Nat Neurosci* 2005; **8**: 1391–400.

179. Kertai, M.D., Whitlock, E.L., and Avidan, M.S. Brain monitoring with electroencephalography and the electroencephalogram-derived bispectral index during cardiac surgery. *Anesth Analg* 2012;**114**:533–46.

180. Kaskinoro, K., Maksimow, A., Långsjö, J., *et al.* Wide inter-individual variability of bispectral index and spectral entropy at loss of consciousness during increasing concentrations of dexmedetomidine, propofol, and sevoflurane. *Br J Anaesth* 2011; **107**: 573–80.

181. Tononi, G. and Edelman, G.M. Consciousness and complexity. *Science* 1998; **282**: 1846–51.

182. Barrett, A.B. and Seth, A.K. Practical measures of integrated information for time-series data. *PLoS Comput Biol* 2011; **7**: e1001052.

183. Massimini, M., Boly, M., Casali, A., *et al.* A perturbational approach for evaluating the brain's capacity for consciousness. *Prog Brain Res* 2009; **177**: 201–14.

184. Barker, A.T., Jalinous, R., and Freeston, I.L. Non-invasive magnetic stimulation of human motor cortex. *Lancet Lond Engl* 1985; **1**: 1106–7.

185. Ilmoniemi, R.J., Virtanen, J., Ruohonen, J., *et al.* Neuronal responses to magnetic stimulation reveal cortical reactivity and connectivity. *Neuroreport* 1997; **8**: 3537–40.

186. Massimini, M., Ferrarelli, F., Huber, R., *et al.* Breakdown of cortical effective connectivity during sleep. *Science* 2005; **309**: 2228–32.

187. Massimini, M., Ferrarelli, F., Esser, S.K., *et al.* Triggering sleep slow waves by transcranial magnetic stimulation. *Proc Natl Acad Sci U S A* 2007; **104**: 8496–501.

188. Funk, C.M., Honjoh, S., Rodriguez, A.V., *et al.* Local slow waves in superficial layers of primary cortical areas during REM sleep. *Curr Biol CB* 2016; **26**: 396–403.

189. Strauss, M., Sitt, J.D., King, J.-R., *et al.* Disruption of hierarchical predictive coding during sleep. *Proc Natl Acad Sci U S A* 2015; **112**: E1353–62.

190. Massimini, M., Ferrarelli, F., Murphy, M., *et al.* Cortical reactivity and effective connectivity during REM sleep in humans. *Cogn Neurosci* 2010; **1**: 176–83.

191. Nieminen, J.O., Gosseries, O., Massimini, M., *et al.* Consciousness and cortical responsiveness: a within-state study during non-rapid eye movement sleep. *Sci Rep* 2016; **6**: 30932.

192. Ferrarelli, F., Massimini, M., Sarasso, S., *et al.* Breakdown in cortical effective connectivity during midazolam-induced loss of consciousness. *Proc Natl Acad Sci U S A* 2010; **107**: 2681–6.

193. Sarasso, S., Boly, M., Napolitani, M., *et al.* Consciousness and complexity during unresponsiveness induced by propofol, xenon, and ketamine. *Curr Biol CB* 2015; **25**: 3099–105.

194. Domino, E.F. Taming the ketamine tiger. *Anesthesiol J Am Soc Anesthesiol* 2010; **113**: 678–84.

195. Collier, B.B. Ketamine and the conscious mind. *Anaesthesia* 1972; **27**: 120–34.

196. Hirota, K. Special cases: ketamine, nitrous oxide and xenon. *Best Pract Res Clin Anaesthesiol* 2006; **20**: 69–79.

197. Oranje, B., van Berckel, B., Kemner, C., *et al.* The effects of a sub-anaesthetic dose of ketamine on human selective attention. *Neuropsychopharmacology* 2000; **22**: 293–302.

198. Watson, T.D., Petrakis, I.L., Edgecombe, J., *et al.* Modulation of the cortical processing of novel and target stimuli by drugs affecting glutamate and GABA neurotransmission. *Int J Neuropsychopharmacol* 2009; **12**: 357–70.

199. Uhrig, L., Janssen, D., Dehaene, S., *et al.* Cerebral responses to local and global auditory novelty under general anesthesia. *NeuroImage* 2016; **141**: 326–40.

200. Casali, A.G., Gosseries, O., Rosanova, M., *et al.* A theoretically based index of consciousness independent of sensory processing and behavior. *Sci Transl Med* 2013; **5**: 198ra105.

201. Harrison, A.H. and Connolly, J.F. Finding a way in: a review and practical evaluation of fMRI and EEG for detection and assessment in disorders of consciousness. *Neurosci Biobehav Rev* 2013; **37**: 1403–19.

202. Peterson, A., Cruse, D., Naci, L., *et al.* Risk, diagnostic error, and the clinical science of consciousness. *NeuroImage Clin* 2015; **7**: 588–97.

203. Giacino, J.T., Ashwal, S., Childs, N., *et al.* The minimally conscious state definition and diagnostic criteria. *Neurology* 2002; **58**: 349–53.

204. Casarotto, S., Comanducci, A., Rosanova, M., *et al.* Stratification of unresponsive patients by an independently validated index of brain complexity. *Ann Neurol* 2016; **80**: 718–29.

205. Gosseries, O., Sarasso, S., Casarotto, S., *et al.* On the cerebral origin of EEG responses to TMS: insights from severe cortical lesions. *Brain Stimulat* 2015; **8**: 142–9.

206. Kübler, A. and Neumann, N. Brain-computer interfaces—the key for the conscious brain locked into a paralyzed body. *Prog Brain Res* 2005; **150**: 513–25.

207. Chaudhary, U., Birbaumer, N., and Ramos-Murguialday, A. Brain-computer interfaces for communication and rehabilitation. *Nat Rev Neurol* 2016; **12**: 513–25.

208. Jarosiewicz, B., Sarma, A.A., Bacher, D., *et al.* Virtual typing by people with tetraplegia using a self-calibrating intracortical brain-computer interface. *Sci Transl Med* 2015; 7: 313ra179.

209. Schiff, N.D., Giacino, J.T., Kalmar, K., *et al.* Behavioural improvements with thalamic stimulation after severe traumatic brain injury. *Nature* 2007; **448**: 600–3.

210. Dobelle, W.H., Mladejovsky, M.G., and Girvin, J.P. Artifical vision for the blind: electrical stimulation of visual cortex offers hope for a functional prosthesis. *Science* 1974; **183**: 440–4.

211. Winkler, R. Elon musk launches Neuralink to connect brains with computers. *Wall Street Journal*. Available at: https://www.wsj.com/articles/ elon-musk-launches-neuralink-to-connect-brains-with-computers-1490642652 (accessed 4 May, 2017).

212. Massimini, M., Ferrarelli, F., Sarasso, S., *et al.* Cortical mechanisms of loss of consciousness: insight from TMS/EEG studies. *Arch Ital Biol* 2012; **150**: 44–55.

213. Pigorini, A., Sarasso, S., Proserpio, P., *et al.* Bistability breaks-off deterministic responses to intracortical stimulation during non-REM sleep. *NeuroImage* 2015; **112**: 105–13.

214. Steriade, M. Arousal: revisiting the reticular activating system. *Science* 1996; **272**: 225–6.

215. Meythaler, J.M., Peduzzi, J.D., Eleftheriou, E., *et al.* Current concepts: diffuse axonal injury-associated traumatic brain injury. *Arch Phys Med Rehabil* 2001; **82**: 1461–71.

216. Murase, N., Duque, J., Mazzocchio, R., *et al.* Influence of interhemispheric interactions on motor function in chronic stroke. *Ann Neurol* 2004; **55**: 400–9.

217. Timofeev, I., Grenier, F., Bazhenov, M., *et al.* Origin of slow cortical oscillations in deafferented cortical slabs. *Cereb Cortex* 2000; **10**(12): 1185–99.

218. Rosanova, M., Fecchio, M., Casarotto, S., *et al.* Sleep-like bistability, loss of causality and complexity in the brain of Unresponsive Wakefulness Syndrome patients. *bioRxiv* Jan. 4, 2018; doi: http://dx.doi.org/10.1101/ 242644.

219. D'Andola, M., Rebollo, B., Casali, A.G., *et al.* Bistability, causality, and complexity in cortical networks: an in vitro perturbational study. *Cereb Cortex* 2017; May 19: 1–10. doi: 10.1093/cercor/bhx122. [Epub ahead of print].

220. Barttfeld, P., Uhrig, L., Sitt, J.D., *et al.* Signature of consciousness in the dynamics of resting-state brain activity. *Proc Natl Acad Sci U S A* 2015; **112**: 887–92.

221. Solovey, G., Alonso, L.M., Yanagawa, T., *et al.* Loss of consciousness is associated with stabilization of cortical activity. *J Neurosci Off J Soc Neurosci* 2015; **35**: 10866–77.

222. Tagliazucchi, E., Chialvo, D.R., Siniatchkin, M., *et al.* Large-scale signatures of unconsciousness are consistent with a departure from critical dynamics. *J R Soc Interface* 2016; **13**: 20151027.

223. Seth, A.K., Barrett, A.B., and Barnett, L. Causal density and integrated information as measures of conscious level. *Philos Trans R Soc Lond Math Phys Eng Sci* 2011; **369**: 3748–67.

224. Marshall, W., Gomez-Ramirez, J., and Tononi, G. Integrated information and state differentiation. *Front Psychol* 2016; **7**: 926.

225. Braun, U., Schäfer, A., Walter, H., *et al.* Dynamic reconfiguration of frontal brain networks during executive cognition in humans. *Proc Natl Acad Sci U S A* 2015; **112**: 11678–83.

226. Oizumi, M., Tsuchiya, N., and Amari, S.-I. Unified framework for information integration based on information geometry. *Proc Natl Acad Sci U S A* 2016; **113**: 14817–22.

227. Tegmark, M. Improved measures of integrated information. *PLoS Comput Biol* 2016; 12(11): e1005123.

228. Zamora-López, G., Chen, Y., Deco, G., *et al.* Functional complexity emerging from anatomical constraints in the brain: the significance of network modularity and rich-clubs. *Sci Rep* 2016; **6**: 38424.

229. Edelman, G. *Bright Air, Brilliant Fire: On The Matter Of The Mind.* Reprint edizione. New York, NY: Basic Books, 1993.

230. Ricard, M. and Singer, W. *Beyond the Self: Conversations between Buddhism and Neuroscience.* Cambridge, MA: MIT Press, 2017.

231. Nagel T. What is it like to be a bat? *Philos Rev* 1974; **83**: 435–50.

232. Descartes, R. *Discourse on Method and Meditations on First Philosophy*, 4th edn. Indianapolis IN: Hackett Publishing Co, Inc, 1998.

233. Montaigne, M., de. *An Apology for Raymond Sebond.* Screech, M.A. (ed.). London : New York, NY: Penguin Classics, 1988.

234. Singer, P. *Animal Liberation: The Definitive Classic of the Animal Movement.* Reissue edition. New York: Harper Perennial Modern Classics, 2009.

235. Edelman, D.B. and Seth, A.K. Animal consciousness: a synthetic approach. *Trends Neurosci* 2009; **32**: 476–84.

236. Mashour, G.A. and Alkire, M.T. Evolution of consciousness: phylogeny, ontogeny, and emergence from general anesthesia. *Proc Natl Acad Sci U S A* 2013; **110**(Suppl. 2): 10357–64.

237. Edelman, D.B., Baars, B.J., and Seth, A.K. Identifying hallmarks of consciousness in non-mammalian species. *Conscious Cogn* 2005; **14**: 169–87.

238. Reiss, D., McCowan, B., and Marino, L. Communicative and other cognitive characteristics of bottlenose dolphins. *Trends Cogn Sci* 1997; **1**: 140–5.

239. Reiss, D. and Marino, L. Mirror self-recognition in the bottlenose dolphin: a case of cognitive convergence. *Proc Natl Acad Sci U S A* 2001; **98**: 5937–42.

240. Pepperberg, I.M. In search of king Solomon's ring: cognitive and communicative studies of Grey parrots (*Psittacus erithacus*). *Brain Behav Evol* 2002; **59**: 54–67.

241. Emery, N.J. and Clayton, N.S. The mentality of crows: convergent evolution of intelligence in corvids and apes. *Science* 2004; **306**: 1903–7.

242. Watanabe, S., Sakamoto, J., Wakita, M. Pigeons' discrimination of paintings by Monet and Picasso. *J Exp Anal Behav* 1995; **63**: 165–74.

243. Mather, J.A. Cephalopod consciousness: behavioural evidence. *Conscious Cogn* 2008; **17**: 37–48.

244. Fiorito, G., Biederman, G.B., Davey, V.A., *et al.* The role of stimulus preexposure in problem solving by *Octopus vulgaris. Anim Cogn* 1998; **1**: 107–12.

245. Montgomery, S. *The Soul of an Octopus: A Surprising Exploration into the Wonder of Consciousness.* Reprint edition. New York, NY: Atria Books, 2016.

246. Anderson, R.C., Mather, J.A., and Wood, J.B. *Octopus: The Ocean's Intelligent Invertebrate.* Portland, OR: Timber Press, 2010.

247. Godfrey-Smith, P. *Other Minds: The Octopus, the Sea, and the Deep Origins of Consciousness.* New York, NY: Farrar, Straus and Giroux, 2016.

248. Loukola, O.J., Perry, C.J., Coscos, L., *et al.* Bumblebees show cognitive flexibility by improving on an observed complex behavior. *Science* 2017; **355**: 833–6.

249. Dyer, F.C. The biology of the dance language. *Annu Rev Entomol* 2002; **47**: 917–49.

250. Cairó, O. External measures of cognition. *Front Hum Neurosci* 2011; **5**: 108.

251. Roth, G. and Dicke, U. Evolution of the brain and intelligence. *Trends Cogn Sci* 2005; **9**: 250–7.

252. Jerison, H.J. The theory of encephalization. *Ann N Y Acad Sci* 1977; **299**: 146–60.

253. Koch, C. and Laurent, G. Complexity and the nervous system. *Science* 1999; **284**: 96–8.

254. Mobbs, P.G. The brain of the honeybee *Apis mellifera*. I. The connections and spatial organization of the mushroom bodies. *Philos Trans R Soc B Biol Sci* 1982; **298**: 309–54.

255. Tononi, G. and Koch, C. Consciousness: here, there and everywhere? *Philos Trans R Soc B Biol Sci* 2015; **370**(1668). pii: 20140167.

256. Silver, D., Huang, A., Maddison, C.J., *et al.* Mastering the game of Go with deep neural networks and tree search. *Nature* 2016; **529**(7587): 484–9.

257. Silver, D., Schrittwieser, J., Simonyan, K., *et al.* Mastering the game of Go without human knowledge. *Nature* 2017; **550**(7676): 354–9.

258. Pfeil, T., Grübl, A., Jeltsch, S., *et al.* Six networks on a universal neuromorphic computing substrate. *Front Neurosci* 2013; **7**: 11.

259. Jarvis, E.D., Güntürkün, O., Bruce, L., *et al.* Avian brains and a new understanding of vertebrate brain evolution. *Nat Rev Neurosci* 2005; **6**: 151–9.

260. Eyal, G., Verhoog, M.B., Testa-Silva, G., *et al.* Unique membrane properties and enhanced signal processing in human neocortical neurons. *eLife* 2016; **5**: pii: e16553.

261. Tegmark, M. Conciousness as a state of matter. *Chaos, Solitons & Fractals* 2015; **76**: 238–70.

262. Wheeler, J.A. *Information, Physics, Quantum: The Search for Links.* Austin, TX: Physics Dept., University of Texas, 1990.

263. Pearl, J. *Causality: Models, Reasoning and Inference*, 2nd edn. Cambridge: Cambridge University Press, 2009.

264. Nelson, C. (2010). Neural Development and Lifelong Plasticity. In D. Keating (Ed.), *Nature and Nurture in Early Child Development* (pp. 45-69). Cambridge: Cambridge University Press. doi:10.1017/CBO9780511975394.003.

265. Innocenti, G.M. and Price, D.J. Exuberance in the development of cortical networks. *Nat Rev Neurosci* 2005; **6**: 955–65.

266. Moore, A.R., Zhou, W.-L., Jakovcevski, I., *et al.* Spontaneous electrical activity in the human fetal cortex in vitro. *J Neurosci Off J Soc Neurosci* 2011; **31**: 2391–8.

267. Shen, J. and Colonnese, M.T. Development of activity in the mouse visual cortex. *J Neurosci Off J Soc Neurosci* 2016; **36**: 12259–75.

268. Penn, A.A. and Shatz, C.J. Brain waves and brain wiring: the role of endogenous and sensory-driven neural activity in development. *Pediatr Res* 1999; **45**: 447–58.

269. Kouider, S., Long, B., Le Stanc, L., *et al.* Neural dynamics of prediction and surprise in infants. *Nat Commun* 2015; **6**: 8537.

270. Gopnik, A., O'Grady, S., Lucas, C.G., *et al.* Changes in cognitive flexibility and hypothesis search across human life history from childhood to adolescence to adulthood. *Proc Natl Acad Sci U S A* 2017; **114**(30).

271. The complete mystical works of Meiser Eckart. Transl. M. O'C Walshe. A Herder & Herder Book. New York, NY: Crossroad Publishing Company, 2010.

272. Mayer-Schonberger, V. and Cukier, K. *Big Data: A Revolution That Will Transform How We Live, Work, and Think.* Boston: Houghton Mifflin, 2013.

INDEX